MULTIPLE MYELOMA:

A Journey of Strength, Courage, and the Never-ending Gift of Hope

Allan G. Osborne

Deborah A. Osborne

SCH Publications

MULTIPLE MYELOMA: A Journey

© 2018 Allan Osborne

DEDICATION

To those who fought and won.
To those who are still fighting.
To those who lost the battle.

Table of Contents

Dedication iii
Preface ix
Part I: An Overview of Multiple Myeloma 1
   1. Multiple Myeloma and How It Develops 3
   2. Symptoms and Diagnosis of Multiple Myeloma 5
   3. Treatments for Multiple Myeloma 7
   4. The Next Steps 11
Part II: The Patient 13
   1. My Diagnosis 15
   2. What Caused My Cancer? 19
   3. My Journey Begins 23
   4. My Journey Continues 27
   5. Maintenance Therapy 31
   6. The New Normal 33
   7. Don't Look Back 37
   8. What Does the Moonshot Initiative Mean for Patients? 39
   9. Have You Heard These? 43
   10. Preventing Multiple Myeloma 47
   11. The Bucket List 51
   12. The Silver Lining 53
   13. Why Not Me? 55
   14. Tips for the Newly Diagnosed 57
   15. Questions to Ask Your Oncologist 61
   16. Is it Chemo Brain or Am I Just Getting Old? 67
   17. The Importance of Clinical Trials 71
   18. Taking Care of Yourself 75

19. Taking Care of Your Caregiver 79

20. The Gift of Time 83

21. Beware of Charlatans Selling Snake Oil 85

Part III: The Caregiver 89

1. In Sickness and in Health 91

2. Multiple Myeloma…What's That? 93

3. Just Breathe… 95

4. Thank you! 97

5. The Tough Question 99

6. November is National Family Caregiver Month 101

7. Diet and Nutrition 103

8. Ask Not… 107

9. Is the Glass Half Full or Half Empty? 109

10. My Tom Brady 111

11. Just a Little More Time 113

12. In the Blink of an Eye 115

13. It's an Honor 117

14. An Inspiration to Us All 119

15. Be Mindful 123

16. Just Let Me Know 125

17. Defining a Clinical Trial and Dispelling Common Misconceptions 129

18. Resources to Help with the High Cost of Medications 133

19. Hold That Thought 137

20. Suggestions for Taking Care of Yourself 139

Part IV: The Promise of the Future: A Reason for Hope 141

1. It's Time to Act 143

2. 2015 Was a Very Good Year 147

3. Trying to Keep It Simple 151

4. What's in the Pipeline? 157

5. Paying it Forward: Why We Volunteer 163

6. Cancer Moonshot – Progress and Promise 167

7. Survival Day 173

Part V: Tributes 177

1. People Come into Your Life for a Reason, a Season or a Lifetime ..179

2. People Who Have Come into My Life 181

3. My Unsung Heroes 185

4. A Tribute to Pat Killingsworth 189

5. This One's for You Joe 191

6. Allan's Medical Team 193

Appendices 197

Appendix 1: Books 199

Appendix 2: Pamphlets, Brochures, and Booklets 205

Appendix 3: Websites 209

Appendix 4: Other Resources 211

Appendix 5: Tips for Evaluating Health Sites on the Internet 213

Preface

We think that when you read something, particularly a book like this one, it is helpful to know something about the authors and their purpose in writing it.

Our story of how we started writing about cancer begins with Allan's diagnosis of multiple myeloma in 2008. Multiple myeloma is a blood cancer that develops in the bone marrow. Up to that point the only knowledge we had of multiple myeloma was that a friend had been diagnosed with the disease approximately twenty years earlier. At that time there were few treatment options and he passed away several months later. Needless to say, we were frightened when given the same diagnosis.

We quickly set out to learn everything possible about the disease, its treatment, and most importantly, its prognosis. Being former educators, we sought out a variety of print and online sources in our research. Even so, we cautiously used the internet, consulting only trusted sites recommended by Allan's oncologist, to find the information we needed to better understand this disease and make informed decisions.

Knowledge is power, and the more we learned about multiple myeloma, the less anxious we felt. In learning all we could about the disease and available treatments, we gained the confidence that although our journey might be difficult, we could successfully navigate through it. Our knowledge gave us a sense of control. It also gave us hope.

As educators and life-long learners we recognized that our quest for knowledge about multiple myeloma needed to continue. To keep updated about the latest research, we began participating in webinars and seminars offered by the Multiple Myeloma Research Foundation (MMRF), the International Myeloma Foundation (IMF), and the Dana-Farber Cancer Institute in Boston. Allan has since been a guest speaker representing the patients' voice at summits sponsored by the MMRF.

Preface

In 2015 we were asked to write monthly blogs for the CoMMunity Gateway section of the MMRF's website. The MMRF is an organization dedicated to finding a cure for this disease. In these blogs, we chronicled our journey and wrote about many aspects of having multiple myeloma. It occurred to us that these blogs could form the basis of a book that others might find useful. So, we have updated and expanded our original blog posts, turning them into longer, more detailed essays. We touch on many subjects and hope that reading them will provide support to other myeloma patients and their caregivers.

This journey is not about our strength or courage but of the strength and courage given to us by the people we have met along the way. It is their inspiration that has given us the gift of never-ending hope.

This book is divided into five parts. Part I presents an overview of multiple myeloma, its diagnosis, and treatment options.

Part II chronicles the journey from Allan's point of view. In the first few chapters he writes about his diagnosis and the various treatments he underwent. In later chapters, he writes about what life with multiple myeloma is like, a life of acceptance and change known as the new normal.

Part III tells the story from the caregiver's point of view. Deb writes about the challenges of having a loved one diagnosed with cancer and what you must do to provide support and care. She offers several essays on the importance of being a caregiver, including basic tips for taking care of yourself while caring for others.

We wrote the chapters in Part IV together. Here we write about some of the major developments that have occurred in the treatment of multiple myeloma over the past few years and some of the promising new treatments that are currently in the pipeline. These developments continue to give us the never-ending gift of hope.

In the final section, Part V, we pay tribute to people who have inspired us and have meant much to us in so many ways. They are people who have given us strength, courage, and the determination to continue to spread awareness and support funding to find a cure.

In the appendices we have assembled lists of resources that we have found to be invaluable in terms of finding accurate, reliable, up-to-date information about multiple myeloma and treatment options. These include books, pamphlets, websites, and seminars that we feel are trusted sources of information.

All royalties from this book will be donated to the MMRF through Team Snug Harbor in the annual Boston Team for Cures 5K Walk/Run.

Our original blogs can be found on the Multiple Myeloma Research Foundation's CoMMunity Gateway at https://community.themmrf.org/. We continue to write blogs for the MMRF and new blogs are posted at the end of each month.

Keep on believing. Life is good.

A.G.O.
D.A.O.

Part I: An Overview of Multiple Myeloma

Overview

1. Multiple Myeloma and How It Develops

Multiple myeloma is a rare blood cancer that develops in the plasma cells found in your bone marrow. Plasma cells are one of the three types of white blood cells in your body. White blood cells help fight infections and disease. Plasma cells produce antibodies critical for maintaining your immune system.

Multiple myeloma develops when healthy plasma cells turn into malignant plasma cells, divide rapidly, and grow out of control. Although the process is complex, genetic abnormalities can turn plasma cells into myeloma cells. When there are too many malignant cells they crowd out normal cells in the bone marrow. Myeloma cells may spread and form tumors in your bones, causing damage to the solid part of the bones. If you only have one tumor it is referred to as a *solitary plasmacytoma*. The label *multiple myeloma* is applied when you have more than one tumor.

> **Multiple myeloma develops when healthy plasma cells turn into malignant plasma cells, divide rapidly, and grow out of control.**

Multiple myeloma can cause several other problems. Patients may develop osteolytic lesions, or soft spots in the bone. This can weaken the bones, leading to fractures. Myeloma patients may experience bone pain, anemia, and kidney problems. Because their immune systems are compromised, myeloma patients are also more susceptible to infections.

More than 90,000 people have multiple myeloma today. Approximately 30,000 new cases are diagnosed each year. Although multiple myeloma is rare, representing just 1% of all cancers, it is the second most common blood cancer. Multiple myeloma is more common among men than women, occurs more often in older individuals, and black Americans are twice as likely to develop myeloma as white Americans.

No definitive cause for multiple myeloma has been found, but there are certain risk factors. In addition to age, gender and race, exposure to radiation or chemicals may pose an increased risk. Being overweight or obese also poses a greater risk of developing myeloma.

There are several subtypes of multiple myeloma. The various subtypes are identified by the kind of protein produced by the myeloma cells. The proteins have heavy and light chains. The heavy chains are identified by letters: A, D, E, G, and M and the light chains are known as kappa and lambda. Most myeloma patients have either the IgG kappa or IgG lambda subtype, followed by IgA or IgA lambda. Other subtypes are rare.

Although multiple myeloma is incurable, it is a treatable disease and the survival rates for myeloma have increased over the last 10 years with the introduction of new treatments. Currently, there are many promising new treatments in clinical trials that are bringing us closer to a cure and improving survival rates even more. The outlook for myeloma patients is improving all the time.

2. Symptoms and Diagnosis of Multiple Myeloma

Some of the more common symptoms of multiple myeloma include anemia, fatigue, bone pain, weakness, excessive thirst, frequent infections, loss of appetite, weight loss, bruising easily, and bleeding easily. Often these symptoms may be attributed to other factors and may not be recognized as signs of multiple myeloma. Many people do not have any symptoms at all.

A variety of tests are used to diagnose multiple myeloma, including routine blood and urine tests. Imaging tests, such as x-rays, CT scans, MRIs, and PET scans may be used. A bone marrow biopsy will confirm the presence and extent of multiple myeloma.

> **A variety of tests are used to diagnose multiple myeloma, including routine blood and urine tests.**

There are three categories of multiple myeloma. The first, monoclonal gammopathy of undetermined significance, usually referred to by its acronym of MGUS, is a condition in which an abnormal protein is present in the blood. MGUS normally does not cause any problems but may be a precursor to myeloma. The second category, smoldering myeloma is asymptomatic and slow growing. It is characterized by increased plasma cells in the bone marrow. Like MGUS, it may not progress to multiple myeloma but needs to be monitored. The final category is active multiple myeloma.

Active myeloma is most commonly staged according to the International Staging System. This system relies on the results of two blood tests, beta-2 microglobulin (ß2-M) and albumin. The stages are:

I: Serum beta-2 microglobulin < 3.5 mg/L and serum albumin ≥ 3.5 g/dL.
II: Neither stage I nor stage III.
III: Serum beta-2 microglobulin ≥ 5.5 mg/L.

An older, but still used, system is known as the Durie-Salmon Staging System. The stages in this system are:

I: A relatively small number of myeloma cells are found. All of the following features must be present:

- Hemoglobin level is only slightly below normal (but still above 10 g/dL)
- Bone x-rays appear normal or show only 1 area of bone damage
- Calcium levels in the blood are normal (less than 12 mg/dL)
- Only a relatively small amount of monoclonal immunoglobulin is in blood or urine

II: A moderate number of myeloma cells are present. Features are between stage I and stage III.

III: A large number of myeloma cells are found. One or more of the following must be present:
- Low hemoglobin level (below 8.5 g/dL)
- High blood calcium level (above 12 mg/dL)
- 3 or more areas of bone destroyed by the cancer
- Large amount of monoclonal immunoglobulin in blood or urine

3. Treatments for Multiple Myeloma

There isn't a single standard treatment protocol for multiple myeloma. A treatment plan will be developed by the patient's medical team based on several factors such as the stage at diagnosis, the subtype of myeloma, and genomic profile. Other factors such as the patient's age and overall health will be taken into consideration. In addition to treatments designed to destroy the myeloma cells, patients may be given therapies to relieve side effects, alleviate symptoms, and respond to complications.

> **In addition to treatments designed to destroy the myeloma cells, patients may be given therapies to relieve side effects, alleviate symptoms, and respond to complications.**

Many patients get a second opinion prior to starting treatment. The doctor giving the second opinion may agree with the first doctor's diagnosis and recommended treatment plan or may suggest other alternatives. Getting a second opinion may give you more information about your options and can make you feel more confident about the decisions that you and your doctor make.

Initially patients may be given radiation to reduce plasmacytomas or tumors. This may then be followed by several cycles of chemotherapy or targeted therapy. This initial treatment is referred to as induction therapy. Patients are often treated with a combination of two or three drugs. A chart listing drugs that are currently approved for the treatment of multiple myeloma is included in Part IV. One commonly used three-drug combination at this time is Revlimid, Velcade, and Decadron, often abbreviated as RVD.

Patients who are good candidates may be given the option of a stem cell transplant. A stem cell transplant begins with high-dose chemotherapy that is very effective in destroying myeloma cells. However, it also kills hematopoietic stem cells in the bone marrow. Hematopoietic stem cells are responsible for forming blood cells. A stem cell transplant replaces those cells. A stem cell transplant often results in a durable remission for multiple myeloma patients. Patients who are not candidates for a stem cell transplant may continue with chemotherapy or targeted therapy for a period of time.

There are two main types of stem cell transplants. One is an autologous transplant in which a patient's own stem cells are harvested and transplanted back following high-dose chemotherapy. An autologous transplant is the type most commonly used to treat multiple myeloma.

In the second type, an allogeneic transplant, a matched donor's stem cells are transplanted into the patient. Donors can be either related or unrelated to the patient. An ideal match would come from an identical twin. An allogeneic transplant carries a higher risk of complications but is effective in treating myeloma.

Patients' stay in the hospital following a stem cell transplant varies but may be for several weeks depending on individual circumstances. The process begins with high-dose chemotherapy followed by the infusion of the stem cells. Several days after the transplant, the transplanted stem cells graft and begin to produce healthy blood cells.

Patients may experience some nausea following the chemotherapy, but this generally can be controlled with medication. Patients will also likely feel fatigued after the chemotherapy but will regain their strength after the stem cells have grafted. At this time the patient is at risk for infections because of the high-dose chemotherapy and for that reason will be in isolation. During this period the patient will be closely monitored by the medical staff so that any problems that may develop can be dealt with immediately.

Following a stem cell transplant, myeloma patients are often put on maintenance medication. The purpose of maintenance therapy is to sustain remission for as long as possible. Research has shown that maintenance medications improve survival.

Unfortunately, as with all powerful drugs, myeloma medications come with some side effects. It is not uncommon for patients to be given other medications, or alternative therapies, to help relieve some of these side effects.

Since your immune system will be compromised and you will be more susceptible to infections, you will likely be given antibiotics and antiviral medications. Your doctor may advise you to avoid crowds and people who are sick. You also may be given some dietary restrictions. If you do get an infection, it should be treated promptly.

Patients who have bone lesions may be given pain medication if needed. Many patients find that acupuncture and massage therapy help to alleviate pain. Patients may also be given bisphosphonates to help strengthen their bones and make them less susceptible to attacks from myeloma cells.

Multiple myeloma and treatments for the disease can cause your blood counts to decrease. If that occurs, you may be given blood transfusions or medications to boost those counts.

The importance of eating properly and getting exercise cannot be overemphasized. It is vital for patients to remain as strong as possible throughout treatment. Even though you may be experiencing a loss of appetite and fatigue, you should try your best to make sure you are getting good nutrition and sufficient exercise. Doing so will help you feel better overall and will go a long way toward helping you to recover faster. Your doctor can refer you to a dietician and exercise physiologist who can help you with this.

Dealing with cancer is stressful. Many patients find it helpful to get some emotional support during this time. Your doctor could refer you to a social worker or therapist who specializes in working with cancer patients. Support groups can also be very helpful. Another option is to talk to someone who has been there. Several "matching" programs exist where newly diagnosed patients are connected with someone who has the same type of cancer. One such program is the One-to-One program at the Dana-Farber Cancer Institute in Boston. Volunteers in these programs are trained to provide support to newly diagnosed patients.

Many patients are given the opportunity to participate in clinical trials. Clinical trials help researchers develop and refine new multiple myeloma treatments. They are necessary for new drugs to become available to all patients. Patients who agree to participate in clinical trials are the first to receive the newest drugs and therapies. They also receive very close monitoring during the trials.

Many new drugs are currently in development and are being evaluated in clinical trials. Some of the more promising ones are discussed in Part IV.

4. The Next Steps

Patients are monitored closely throughout treatment to see if the therapies are working. During this time, many of the same tests that were given to diagnose the disease will be repeated. Since multiple myeloma is an incurable disease, it is important for patients to be closely monitored even after they have finished treatment.

> **Since multiple myeloma is an incurable disease, it is important for patients to be closely monitored even after they have finished treatment.**

One of the tests doctors frequently use to measure the degree of myeloma in a patient is known as the M-spike. The M-spike measures the monoclonal proteins in the blood. Monoclonal proteins are abnormal, and unneeded, antibodies produced by myeloma cells.

A patient's response to myeloma treatment is generally classified in one of the following categories: Molecular complete response, immunophenotypic complete response, stringent complete response, complete response, near complete response, very good partial response, partial response, minimal response, stable disease, or progressive disease. Classification is based on several factors including the amount of monoclonal proteins in the blood, the percent of plasma cells in the bone marrow, and the degree of bone disease.

The term *minimal residual disease*, abbreviated as MRD, means that there are only a few myeloma cells remaining when a patient has achieved a complete response or better. Blood, bone marrow, and urine tests are used to ascertain MRD, but more sensitive tests are in development. With these new tests, myeloma experts hope to be able to detect the complete absence of myeloma, known as MRD-0.

If the myeloma is not responsive to a particular therapy, it is referred to as being refractory. Some patients may not respond to certain therapies and in others a treatment that appeared to be working may become refractory. If patients relapse quickly after their initial therapy their disease is also considered to be refractory. When patients are refractory they may have new drugs added to their treatment regimen or may be given an entirely new combination of drugs. This is referred to as second-line therapy.

Despite all the advances that have been made in the past few years, multiple myeloma is still an incurable disease and patients may experience a relapse after a period of remission. If a patient relapses after a sustained period of remission, they may be treated again with the same therapies they initially received, or an entirely new regimen may be tried.

Sources

The following sources were used to obtain information for this section. Their websites can be consulted for further information.
- American Cancer Society, www.cancer.org
- Multiple Myeloma Research Foundation, www.themmrf.org
- National Cancer Institute, www.cancer.gov

Part II: The Patient

The Patient

1. My Diagnosis

As we had planned, in July 2008 my wife and I retired after very rewarding careers in education. Life was good, and, although we had loved our jobs, we were very excited to be entering the next phase of our lives. Like many newly-retired people, we started working on home improvement projects, making travel plans, and talking about all the things we wanted to do in our retirement.

One of our projects was to convert a spare bedroom into what we call the reading room. It's a place to relax, listen to soft music, and read. In mid-October, while hanging some new curtains, instead of going down two flights of stairs to get a stepladder, I just grabbed a convenient chair. I fell as I stepped off the chair and injured my back. I wasn't concerned because I thought that I had just sprained it a bit. That night I took two ibuprofens and used a heating pad on it.

When the back pain wasn't any better after a couple of days, I went to see my primary care physician, who thought it was just a pulled muscle. He told me to continue with the ibuprofen and heating pad, but to call him in a week if it still wasn't better and he'd order an MRI. Well, it got worse rather than better, so my doctor sent me for the MRI. I still wasn't concerned. I figured the worst it could be was a herniated disk. Boy was I wrong.

Right after getting the MRI we left for a trip to San Antonio to attend a conference of the Education Law Association, an organization I had been involved with for many years. During a layover in Houston I checked my messages and there were several, on both my home and cell phones, from my physician asking me to call him right away. When I reached him, he didn't want to give me the news over the phone but, since I was so far away, he had no choice. He informed me that the MRI indicated that I had a tumor on my spine that appeared to be malignant and was consistent with one that had spread from somewhere else. I was stunned. I had never expected that. I think Deb was even more stunned.

My doctor tried to reassure me by telling me that it didn't make sense to him. I had all the cancer screenings I should have had, such as colonoscopies and PSAs, and nothing had ever even hinted at cancer.

Nevertheless, he told me that I needed to come home immediately to see an oncologist. I think the gravity of the situation really hit home when I heard the word oncologist. When I realized that I could possibly have cancer, I was frightened.

We arranged to come home the next day. My doctor had set up an appointment with a local oncologist for the following day. Even though we have flown to many distant places, the plane ride back to Boston seemed like the longest we had ever taken. It was an eternity. Neither of us slept much that night. We spent a good part of the next day gathering the MRI plates and my medical records. Our anxiety was at an all-time high when we entered the oncologist's office a day later.

The oncologist, a wonderful and extremely compassionate professional, immediately put us at ease. He explained that it was the radiologist's job to get us to his office, and thus had to alert us to the worst-case scenario. After looking at the MRI he said it looked like a plasmacytoma to him. He explained what a plasmacytoma was but assured us that, although serious, it could be treated successfully. He ordered comprehensive blood tests and a full body scan. We met with him the next day and he informed us that the tests did not show any sign of cancer in any other organs. He then sent us to Brigham and Women's Hospital in Boston to consult with an orthopedic surgeon and to have the tumor on my spine biopsied.

The biopsy results indicated that the tumor on my spine was, as the oncologist suspected, a plasmacytoma. The good news was that it was a solitary plasmacytoma and that it could be dealt with via radiation rather than surgery. However, the fact that it was a plasmacytoma meant that multiple myeloma was suspected.

As explained in Part I, multiple myeloma is a blood cancer that forms in the plasma cells found in bone marrow. The only time I had heard of multiple myeloma was twenty years earlier when the husband of a good friend and colleague was diagnosed with the disease and passed away several months later. When I heard the term *multiple myeloma* my heart stopped, and I must have turned white. The oncologist instantly recognized my fear and quickly explained that many advances had recently been made in the treatment of multiple myeloma so that it was now treated as a chronic disease. He added that many patients with this disease, including some of his, lived for fifteen or twenty years and with the new therapies even longer remissions were possible. He assured me that if I did indeed have multiple myeloma, it could be treated successfully. He provided me with some brochures that gave me more hope.

Blood tests and a bone marrow biopsy confirmed that I had multiple myeloma. Luckily, we had caught it early. The biopsy and serum protein tests indicated that I had stage II myeloma. Thanks to falling off that chair (which now holds a place of honor in our household), an early diagnosis, and having a great medical team, the prognosis was very good.

> A bone marrow biopsy confirmed that I had multiple myeloma. Luckily, we had caught it early.

As I look back, I can't help but think how lucky I was. If I had not fallen off that chair, perhaps several more months would have gone by before the multiple myeloma was detected and the disease may have been more advanced. I am also fortunate that my primary care physician, who is very patient-oriented, did not follow the wishes of insurance companies that do not recommend having MRIs for every little back pain a patient might have. Instead of sending me for physical therapy, as another doctor might have, he ordered the test. I am also fortunate that he sent me to a highly competent oncologist who had experience with multiple myeloma.

Naturally, once given the diagnosis I wanted to know everything I could about multiple myeloma. My oncologist, however, cautioned against turning to the internet, explaining that much of what I would find on the information superhighway about myeloma was either incorrect or outdated. He told me that one good place to find accurate information was the National Institute of Health. I have also found two other reliable sources of information in the websites of the Multiple Myeloma Research Foundation and the International Myeloma Foundation. Both organizations are leaders in promoting and funding research in multiple myeloma. Their websites are updated constantly and contain current information about treatments and research results.

My oncologist's advice about websites being outdated was on target and still holds true today. So many advances have been made in this field in the past five years that any website that is not constantly updated does not contain reliable, accurate information. For example, the survival rates for myeloma patients listed on many websites are rather gloomy. But they are not true. These survival statistics are several years old. To put it bluntly, most of us walking around today with multiple myeloma have already surpassed the survival data listed in many web sites. Survival predictions today are much more optimistic and are getting better all the time. In fact, since so many therapies are still in their infancy, those of us being treated today are creating new survival statistics.

The best advice I have for newly diagnosed myeloma patients is to not panic. Yes, any cancer diagnosis is scary and there is never a good time to get cancer. Even so, with all the advances that have been made in treating multiple myeloma, the prognosis is better than it has ever been, and it is getting better all the time. We have every reason to hope for, and expect, many years of remission and even a cure. As you read the essays in this book, I hope you will see why I sign off with the motto "Life is good" and Deb ends hers with the phrase "Don't stop believing."

Life is good.

2. What Caused My Cancer?

*"Felt an emptiness inside to which he just could not relate
Brought on by a simple twist of fate."*
Bob Dylan, 1975
Simple Twist of Fate

After being diagnosed with multiple myeloma I wanted to know what I had done wrong to cause this cancer. I wasn't a smoker and I drank moderately. Although I certainly could stand to lose a couple of pounds, I wasn't too overweight. I had always tried to live a healthy lifestyle by eating properly and keeping fit. I also saw my physician regularly and had all tests that he recommended, so getting the diagnosis came as a complete surprise.

With my family history, I was more concerned about heart disease, stroke, or Alzheimer's disease. My father had heart disease most of his life and passed away from complications of a third stroke at the age of 82. My mother died from complications of early onset Alzheimer's disease at the age of 72. Thus, cancer was not something I worried about.

When I asked my oncologist what caused multiple myeloma, he answered simply, "Bad luck." He went on to explain that there were some theories but nothing definitive. He assured me that I had not done anything to cause my cancer. To paraphrase Mr. Dylan, this disease that was giving me that empty feeling inside to which I just could not relate, was brought on by a simple twist of fate.

> **To paraphrase Mr. Dylan, this disease that was giving me that empty feeling inside to which I just could not relate, was brought on by a simple twist of fate.**

Multiple myeloma is more common in males, African-Americans, and those over 65. Although it does not have a hereditary link, having a family member with multiple myeloma does increase your chances. Other possible risk factors include excessive exposure to radiation, obesity, and having another plasma cell disorder. I was a 57-year-old white male with no history of it in my family. Other than dental x-rays I had almost no exposure to radiation, was not obese, and did not have any other blood disease. I only had one risk factor – I was a male.

While my oncologist's reassurance that I had not done anything to cause my cancer was comforting, the bad luck explanation also did not fit. Why? Throughout my life, I have always been blessed with good luck. I was lucky to be born into a great family. I had the advantage of a good education. Right out of college I landed a job that evolved into a very rewarding career. I was also lucky because I had found my perfect mate and had a wonderful marriage. That turned out to be the best luck of all.

Not being ready to accept the prospect that perhaps my luck had turned, I started to investigate the theories of what caused multiple myeloma. I knew it wouldn't change anything, but my intellectual curiosity made me want to know more. Also, I felt that if I had done something to cause this disease, then I needed to stop doing it.

I did not find any definitive information about possible causes of multiple myeloma. Statistics showing that workers in agriculture, leather industries, cosmetology, and petroleum industries have a higher incidence of multiple myeloma than the general population suggest that exposure to certain chemicals may be one possible cause. In particular, heavy metals, herbicides, insecticides, hair dyes, petroleum products, and asbestos may be culprits.

The chemical exposure theory is bolstered by the fact that responders to the September 11th attacks also have a higher incidence of multiple myeloma. Recent studies have also associated exposure to Agent Orange, a defoliant used during the Vietnam War, to multiple myeloma. Other studies show a correlation between exposure to DDT, a once commonly-used insecticide, to myeloma. Although the research and statistics are not definitive, they do suggest a possible link.

So, how do I fit into this? Being an avid gardener, I have used chemical fertilizers, insecticides, and herbicides most of my life. I also worked in a hardware store that sold these products and I handled them extensively. In addition, for years one of my hobbies has been photography. When I was younger I had a photographic darkroom in my cellar that was not well-ventilated. Since I spent a fair amount of time there, I did breathe in more than my fair share of photographic chemicals.

Did this exposure cause my multiple myeloma? I don't really know, but just to be safe I now make a concerted effort to limit my exposure to chemicals. I still spend much of my leisure time outside working on the lawn and garden. Now, however, I try to use organic products as much as I can. When I must use chemicals, I take precautions by wearing a mask and washing up immediately after using them. We also hire professionals to do any spraying. I have also made the transition from film to digital photography.

Will this help to reduce my chance of a recurrence of multiple myeloma? Again, who knows? But it won't hurt. And it may even help to prevent me from getting other illnesses associated with chemical exposure. As you will see from reading these essays, I am a firm believer that living a healthy lifestyle has had much to do with my remission.

Life is good.

The Patient

3. My Journey Begins

Once anyone receives a diagnosis of cancer, I think most of us are anxious for treatment to begin. Although we are apprehensive, and don't quite know what to expect, we want to begin attacking those cancer cells right away. We don't want them in our bodies and the sooner we eliminate them the better.

My oncologist gave us some excellent advice. He explained that there would be several steps in the treatment process, but we would take it one step at a time. He cautioned us to not get ahead of ourselves by thinking too much about the next step. Rather than worry about what was to come, he told us that we needed to focus on what was happening in the present.

Many people with multiple myeloma, particularly those who were diagnosed in advanced stages, have significant bone problems, such as lesions or even fractures. I was fortunate that I did not have any serious bone involvement, but I did have a plasmacytoma on my spine that caused considerable pain and interfered with my ability to walk. A plasmacytoma is a tumor consisting of malignant plasma cells that accumulate in either the bones or soft tissues.

Fortunately, I did not require surgery and we could treat the plasmacytoma with radiation. The whole process was straightforward. Each treatment lasted only a couple of minutes. In fact, with my mobility problems, it took me longer to get up on the table than it took the technician to administer the radiation. The radiation treatment consisted of two brief blasts – one from my back and one from my side.

The pain lessened with each radiation session until it was gone completely. But the treatment caused some fatigue that increased as we went along. How could two short blasts of radiation cause me to feel so tired? The radiation oncologist explained that it was because my body was working hard to recover from the effects of the radiation. When the cancer cells were killed, some good cells were also destroyed. My body worked hard to repair them, and this caused the fatigue.

My last session of radiation was bittersweet. I was certainly glad that it was over. Even though I had only had ten sessions, I became quite attached to the radiation oncologist and her team. I have the habit of getting attached to people who do things to save my life. The radiation oncologist was a very positive person who helped me to better understand my situation and prognosis. The two radiation technicians were very kind and offered me much encouragement. That final session was emotional for me because these people supported me during the first step of my treatment and I was sad that they would now be out of my life.

Once the radiation was over I was anxious to begin chemotherapy and was disappointed to learn that I had to take a break to recover from the radiation. That did make sense, but I wasn't happy about it. I wanted to begin to kill those cancer cells right away. I didn't like the idea that they were swimming around in my bloodstream looking for places to wreak havoc.

My chemotherapy regimen was fairly new at that time but is now standard. I had six three-week cycles of Revlimid, Velcade, and dexamethasone (RVD), two weeks on followed by one week off. In 2009, Velcade was administered intravenously but now may be injected subcutaneously. Revlimid, also known as lenalidomide, is an immunomodulatory drug that acts by stimulating your immune system to fight your cancer. Velcade or bortezomib is a proteasome inhibitor that works by preventing cancer cells from growing, dividing, and multiplying. Dexamethasone is a corticosteroid that in high doses can kill myeloma cells. It also helps the Revlimid to be more effective. Since myeloma can attack your bones, once a month I also got Zometa, a bone-strengthening medication.

I have always hated needles, especially those that are inserted into a vein. The head IV nurse recognized this right away. I'm not quite sure how she knew. Maybe it was the look of fear on my face or the clenched teeth. To make things easier for me, she used a smaller needle, normally used for infants, which she referred to as the "baby needle." I didn't care what she called it, if it hurt less.

All the people who cared for me in the oncologist's office during those eighteen weeks were wonderful. The IV nurse teased me about needing the baby needle but was very gentle and reassuringly held my hand as she inserted it. Another was the nurse practitioner who oversaw the whole chemo process. They are both very special people and I don't think I could have gotten through the chemo without them. The technician who drew my blood and the front desk receptionists were super people who did everything they could to make the process easier. I wasn't just another patient in their office. I felt like the really cared about me.

In early March, when I was about half way through the chemo, my oncologist told us that during the next week off, he wanted us to go away to someplace warm. We booked a quick trip to San Juan where we spent five days just relaxing. Once again, my oncologist's advice was right on target. It was just what we needed. We came back feeling refreshed and ready for the next couple of cycles.

Overall the chemo went well. I did develop some neuropathy in my feet and we had to reduce the Velcade for the final cycle. I had the usual side effects from the Revlimid, but nothing I couldn't live with. As far as I was concerned, the only side effect I had from the dexamethasone was that it kept me awake at night on the day I took it. However, my wife might tell a different story. She felt that I was a very different person on the dex. I guess I was a bit argumentative at times and a bit difficult to get along with. The first couple of doses of Zometa gave me some mild flu-like symptoms for a day, but after that it just made me tired.

I met some inspirational people during my treatment. When you are in the chemo room connected to an IV for several hours at a time, you have the opportunity to speak to other patients. Those conversations allowed us to develop a special comradery. We encouraged each other and celebrated each other's milestones.

At the end of my final cycle I had another bone marrow biopsy. A few days later my oncologist called to tell me that the biopsy showed that the chemo had done its job. Remission is the most beautiful word in the English language.

> **My oncologist called to tell me that the biopsy showed that the chemo had done its job. Remission is the most beautiful word in the English language.**

All things considered, I have to say that the entire chemotherapy treatment went well. The results speak for themselves. I think that following my oncologist's advice to take things one step at a time helped me to get through the chemo. Throughout the process I never thought about what would come next. Instead, I focused on what I wanted for a final result.

That was not the end of the treatment. Since multiple myeloma is incurable, it was likely that some cancerous cells remained. Although none had been detected, that did not mean they were not there. The tests that were available at that time were not sophisticated enough to detect all myeloma cells. While I had responded to the chemo, we decided to investigate the possibility of a stem cell transplant to ensure a longer remission. That would be the next part of the journey.

Life is good.

4. My Journey Continues

In the previous essays I chronicled my diagnosis and the initial steps in my treatment. In this chapter, I continue the journey by writing about my experience with a stem cell transplant.

Deb and I are volunteers in the One-to-One program at the Dana-Farber Cancer Institute in Boston. In this program, we are paired with newly diagnosed patients and their caregivers to provide support as they move through the treatment process. Many of the people we coach in this program are facing a stem cell transplant. At the very least they are apprehensive. Some are downright scared. I am sharing my experience in the hope that I can ease those concerns and fears for those of you who are facing a stem cell transplant.

To begin the process my oncologist sent us to Dana-Farber for a consult with a transplant specialist to see if I was a good candidate for the procedure. The specialist agreed with my oncologist that I was an excellent candidate because of the good response I had to the induction chemo. Even though test results showed that I was in remission, both doctors felt that we should go the transplant route to eliminate any residual disease that still existed. I didn't need convincing. Something inside me told me that this was the way to go.

> **I didn't need convincing. Something inside me told me that this was the way to go.**

A stem cell transplant is a complicated process with many steps. Although both doctors felt that I was a good candidate, I still needed several more tests, and the most comprehensive physical exam I have ever had, to make sure that I was otherwise healthy enough for the transplant.

Once I was cleared for the transplant, Deb and I met with a transplant nurse who went over the whole process step-by-step. She was very thorough in her explanation, and answered all our questions, so that we were very clear as to what to expect. She also gave us a binder that provided us with comprehensive information about the procedure and what we had to do at each step. We refer to that binder as the "rule book" because it clearly let us know what I could and could not do during the next few months. The binder was so comprehensive we knew that it could be overwhelming. We decided to approach it the way we approached the whole treatment process – to take it one step at a time. We read one section at a time and would not move on to the next section until we were sure that we fully understood what we had just read.

To begin the process, I was given a high dose infusion of Cytoxan, a powerful chemotherapy agent that is used to treat many cancers. It works by interfering with a cancer cell's ability to divide and replicate itself. I did experience some side effects from the Cytoxan, most notably I lost most of my hair. I also had some minor nausea, fatigue, and lost my appetite for a few days.

Since I was having an autologous transplant, the next step was to harvest my own stem cells. The collection was preceded by 10 days of injections of a growth agent to ensure that I would have abundant stem cells to harvest. I also had a Hickman catheter installed to make the procedure easier. The collection of stem cells took place over two days. During these two days I was tethered to a machine that extracted my blood, removed the stem cells, and then returned my blood.

I was admitted to the hospital a few days after the collection. I was given two more days of high dose chemo – this time Melphalan. Melphalan is another powerful chemotherapy that works by stopping the growth of cancer cells. I did experience some nausea from the Melphalan, but the nurses gave me medication to control it. After taking the Melphalan I was quite fatigued and didn't have much of an appetite. I also lost the rest of my hair.

The third day was transplant day. I didn't know what to expect but I anticipated that the world's greatest doctors would converge on my room to give me the transplant. Instead a nurse came in with a bag containing a putrid-looking substance and announced, "I've got your stem cells." After checking and double checking everything with a second nurse, she connected me to some monitoring equipment and attached the bag to my IV. I don't remember how long it took, but it was over very quickly.

The next few days were somewhat of a blur. I remember sleeping much of the time. My blood counts kept going down, but the doctors assured me that this was what was supposed to happen. I was given some infusions of blood products. Then several days later the blood counts started going up, which meant that the stem cells had grafted.

One of the nasty side effects of the chemo is mouth sores. To help prevent them, I was given an oral hygiene routine to follow. As part of that routine every two hours I had to alternately use one of two different types of mouthwash. There were times, particularly when I felt nauseous, that I really didn't want to do this. Still, I forced myself to follow this routine without fail. I didn't get the mouth sores. Sticking to this routine is no guarantee that you won't get mouth sores; however, failing to follow it may very well result in sores.

Every day I got stronger, but I still slept quite a bit. Even so, there was plenty of activity in my room. Every morning a team of oncologists, residents, and physician's assistants came in to examine me. The nurses checked on me frequently. Nurse assistants were in often to check my vital signs. I felt very assured that if anything went wrong, my medical team would be right there to take care of it.

Altogether, I spent 18 days in the hospital, but it really hadn't seemed that long. Perhaps that was because I had slept through much of it. Nevertheless, it was good to be home.

Following the transplant my immune system was very compromised. Consequently, to prevent infection, during the next 90 days I was in isolation and had some dietary restrictions. I couldn't eat anything raw and could only have meals that were prepared inside my own house. Although I was in isolation and couldn't be in crowds, I was able to go outside and have a few visitors as long as they were healthy and wore masks. After the 90 days were up, the dietary restrictions were gradually reduced, but I still needed to take precautions to avoid infection, particularly because we were at the height of flu season.

Exercise was an important aspect of my overall recovery. I walked every day and continued to get stronger each day. Deb and I enjoy gardening and the worst restriction I had was not being able to work in the yard that summer. That fall, however, my oncologist gave me permission to rake leaves if I wore a mask. I always hated to rake leaves but was never so glad to be able to do so.

The best piece of advice I have for anyone facing a transplant is to follow your doctors' orders religiously. They know what they are doing and there is a reason for all their instructions. Deb and I are rule-followers and did what we were told. The process went smoothly, and we did not encounter any serious problems. We credit that to having strictly followed the doctors' orders.

As I look back, if I ever must have another transplant, I won't be too happy about it, but I won't hesitate to do it. I won't say that it was easy, and these certainly weren't the best days of my life, but the end result was worth it.

As I write this, I am now almost nine years post-transplant with an M-spike of 0 and all other test results are where they ought to be. My overall health is very good. I can do everything I want to do. I might do it a bit slower than I used to, but that is due more to the fact that I am getting older, not that I have multiple myeloma.

Life is good.

5. Maintenance Therapy

Shortly after I had recovered from my stem cell transplant my oncologist talked to me about a clinical trial investigating the benefits of post-transplant maintenance therapy with Revlimid. The theory was that since either a transplant or continuous treatment with Revlimid showed benefits in terms of progression-free survival, wouldn't a combination be even better? It made sense to me and I was interested.

Unfortunately, the clinical trials were closed. However, a few months later they were ended early because the results had been so positive. So, at that time, based on the results of the clinical trials, we decided that maintenance therapy was the way to go for me. The regimen consisted of 10 mg daily, 21 days on, followed by seven days off.

I was very lucky in two respects. First, the Revlimid did the trick and kept my multiple myeloma in remission. Second, I tolerated it very well. I did have a few side effects, such as fatigue (particularly during the third week of the cycle), gastrointestinal problems, and some minor neuropathy. However, the side effects were nothing I couldn't live with. The way I saw it, they were a small price to pay for being alive.

> **However, the side effects were nothing I couldn't live with. The way I saw it, they were a small price to pay for being alive.**

After I was on the maintenance therapy for a couple of years my oncologist spoke to me about research that had shown there was a slight risk of developing secondary cancers from Revlimid, particularly for those of us who had been given Melphalan prior to transplant. Even so, the risk appeared to be small and needed to be considered in light of the fact that without the maintenance therapy, a relapse of the myeloma was more likely. We decided the benefits of maintenance therapy outweighed the risk and I stayed on it.

After being on maintenance therapy for five years, I asked my oncologist what he thought about reducing the dosage to 5 mg. After much thought, he said he agreed, and even added that he would be comfortable with me coming off it totally. My numbers were all fine:

protein and IGG counts were normal, light chains were well within the average range, and there was no detectable M-spike. I wasn't yet ready to take the plunge and go completely off Revlimid, so we decided to continue, but with the lower dose.

After a year on the lower dose, my test results had not changed. There was still no sign of myeloma. I had seen a slight - but for the most part insignificant - reduction in the side effects. I again had the discussion with my oncologist about coming off Revlimid completely. Now the benefit vs. risk equation had changed. At this point, there was no data about the long-term side effects of Revlimid maintenance for the simple reason that very few patients had been on it long-term. On the other hand, my chance of a relapse, while ever-present, seemed low.

Since Revlimid maintenance is still in its infancy, there are many unanswered questions. Is there any survival benefit to staying on Revlimid for many years? Does the chance of developing a secondary cancer increase the longer you are on Revlimid? Will going off Revlimid increase the chance of a relapse? Are there other long-term side effects we don't even know about? Researchers are working on answers to these and many other questions. Based on the data they have available, the prevalent thinking among the experts is that most myeloma patients should stay on maintenance therapy until progression.

With the information available, I had to decide if I was ready to come off Revlimid and fly solo? I decided that I was. I was willing to take the risk and was confident that it was the right thing to do. I was also reassured by the fact that my medical team would keep a very close eye on me. Since coming off Revlimid, my test results have been stable, but I know that if they start to head in the wrong direction, my decision can be reversed.

This clearly is not right for everyone, particularly since current research shows that there is a survival benefit with long-term Revlimid therapy. As my oncologist explained to me, 98 percent of myeloma patients should continue with maintenance therapy. But, he feels that I fall into the 2 percent who will do fine without it. As Deb says, "It's always an adventure."

Life is good.

6. The New Normal

When I talk to newly diagnosed multiple myeloma patients, one of the comments I hear most often is, "I just want to get back to normal." When I hear that I cringe a bit because I know that, no matter what, their lives will never go back to what was normal. Instead they will experience what is known as the new normal.

Just exactly what is the new normal? Well, it just means that your life is going to be different. But it doesn't mean that it is going to be worse. It means you may have to make some adjustments and some lifestyle changes. But, it also means that some aspects of your life will be better.

> Just exactly what is the new normal? Well, it just means that your life is going to be different. But it doesn't mean that it is going to be worse.

The new normal will mean frequent doctors' visits with blood tests. Even after the initial phases of your treatment are over, it is likely that you will be on some type of maintenance regimen. That, of course, means that you will still take medication with all the side effects that go along with it.

There is a positive side to the new normal as well. On balance, I think the positive aspects of the new normal far outweigh the negative aspects. It sounds like a cliché, but you really do appreciate the little things in life after this experience. You will also make many new friends in the myeloma community and you will cherish their friendship.

The new normal does, however, require some adjustments. Here are a few things that I have found have helped me to adapt to my new lifestyle.

The first step is acceptance. You need to accept the fact that life will be different. Throughout our lives, we often must make some adjustments. We change jobs. Our personal and domestic situations change. We are getting older and can't do all the things we used to do. All require lifestyle adjustments. Adjusting to the new normal is no different.

Maintaining a positive attitude is very important. Several weeks ago, I met a myeloma patient who maintains a list of all the positive things in his life. He adds one thing to his list every day. Doing this keeps him focused on the fact that although his life is different, it is good.

Having a good support system in place is very beneficial. Although I have found that most people are very understanding when it comes to the changes I need to make in my overall lifestyle, there are a few people who just don't get it. It makes the adjustments much easier when your friends and family, not only understand, but help you in making the changes you need to make. When friends don't understand, you need to educate them.

I think the hardest part of the new normal is dealing with the changes that occur because of the disease itself and the side effects of the medications we take. Most of us who have myeloma, even when it's in remission, will have compromised immune systems, and will experience medication side effects such as fatigue that affect how we live our lives.

We have not become germophobic – but Deb and I are very conscientious in trying to avoid bacteria and viruses. We both worked in school systems where we were exposed to all sorts of viruses and infections. We built up good immune systems, but mine was completely lost because of my myeloma and its treatment. Now we must avoid people who are sick. We use hand sanitizer constantly. When we travel, we bring along disinfectant towelettes to wipe down the trays and armrests on planes and everything we might touch in hotel rooms. We take these precautions when we travel so that we can enjoy our trips without me getting sick.

I think the fatigue was the side effect that was the hardest for me. I've always been an active person and found it difficult to pace myself so that I didn't get overtired. But I learned. Now, we're very careful to not schedule too many social engagements in one week. Pacing ourselves, and sometimes saying no to invitations, helps me to not only stay healthy, but better enjoy the things I do.

In the same way, it's important to set realistic expectations. Try to understand what you can and cannot do. If necessary, set new goals and work on them. If you are no longer able to do something you enjoy doing, develop a new interest. Perhaps you have always wanted to take up a new hobby but never had the time to invest in it. Now is as good a time as ever to explore that interest.

Finally, celebrate the small things and take the time to enjoy what you have.

I sign off on each of my essays with the phrase, "Life is good." Yes, life is different now. But it's good. It's very good. In fact, it's fantastic!

7. Don't Look Back

"Shake the dust off of your feet, don't look back."

Bob Dylan, 1980
Pressing On

When I was the principal of an elementary school I was fortunate enough to work with a great assistant principal. Bob and I complimented each other well because we each had different skills and strengths. However, we shared two things: We were both Bob Dylan fans and we both believed in the "don't look back" philosophy.

"Don't look back" meant that we never beat ourselves up if decisions we made turned out to not have been the best course of action. If we thought we had made the right decision at the time, but it turned out otherwise, we took Mr. Dylan's advice and shook the dust off our feet and moved on. We never lamented, "Gee, I wish we had done this instead."

However, "don't look back" did not mean that we didn't learn from our mistakes. In fact, one of Bob's strengths was his ability to analyze situations post hoc to figure out what went right or wrong. Our analysis was always future-oriented with the purpose of figuring out a better way to handle a similar situation next time. We did not say, "This is what we should have done," but rather, said, "This is what we'll do next time."

The don't look back philosophy has served me well in my journey through multiple myeloma. Along the way, we have many decisions to make involving the choice of a doctor, the best treatment options, taking other steps to improve our overall health, and, perhaps most importantly, how to maximize our overall quality of life. We treat these decisions as though they are matters of life and death for a simple reason – many of them are.

> **The don't look back philosophy has served me well in my journey through multiple myeloma.**

In a post on the MMRF's CoMMunity Gateway, a fellow myeloma patient, the late Pat Killingsworth, wrote about the steps he took when faced with an important decision about his treatment. In that post he stressed the importance of getting all the information you can and relying on the expert opinions of your medical team. As Pat indicated, that's easy when your doctors all agree, but puts the onus on you if they have divergent thoughts.

I have two oncologists. One is a local specialist who gave me my initial diagnosis, administered my chemotherapy, and coordinates all of my follow-up care. The second is a stem cell transplant specialist who handled that portion of my treatment and continues with follow-up monitoring. I am fortunate that these two doctors are in constant contact and have always agreed about the best course of action. Throughout most of my journey, I have had few decisions because these two experts told me what they thought we should do and I never questioned their advice.

There was, however, a major decision that was left up to me. That was the decision I wrote about previously – the decision to go off maintenance Revlimid. Although both doctors agreed that it was a good move, they made it clear that the decision was mine. Time will tell whether that was the right decision or not. But I am sure of one thing: I will not look back. If I relapse I will not bemoan that decision and say, "I never should have stopped taking Revlimid." My doctors gave me a recommendation based on their expert knowledge and experience. I have the utmost confidence in both oncologists and took that advice because I had a gut feeling that it was right.

I don't waste time or mental energy worrying about whether it is the right course of action. If I relapse I also won't waste time or mental energy wondering if I would have done better if I had continued with the maintenance therapy. Instead, I'll dig out Dylan's *Saved* CD, put my headphones on, and listen to him sing *Pressing On*. Then I'll shake the dust off my feet and make the next decision about my treatment, using whatever new knowledge I have gained from my experience. Rather than dwell on my past, I prefer to focus on my future. The future is too short to live it with regrets.

Life is good.

8. What Does the Moonshot Initiative Mean for Patients?

In his final State of the Union address President Obama announced what has become known as the "Moonshot" initiative to cure cancer. This initiative was headed up by Vice President Biden. The Vice President, who lost his son to brain cancer in 2015, is all too aware of the need for the federal government to step up its efforts to coordinate and financially support research that will lead to a cure.

President Obama is not the first Chief Executive to declare war on cancer. In his 1971 State of the Union address President Nixon stated that the time had come "when the same kind of concentrated effort that split the atom and took man to the moon should be turned toward conquering this dread disease." Later that year he signed the National Cancer Act, strengthening the National Cancer Institute and increasing funding for cancer research. Although cancer is still with us 45 years later, significant breakthroughs have been made. Consequently, while there were only three million cancer survivors in 1971, today there are over twelve million of us.

President Obama's Moonshot initiative represented a step forward in the war on cancer. In his final year in office, Vice President Biden focused on two objectives. First, he worked to increase both public and private resources to fight cancer. Second, he took steps to break down the barriers that existed so that researchers could work together and share information. The Vice President and his staff worked with leading cancer researchers to formulate plans on how this could be accomplished.

Can this work? I believe it can. In many respects, this model sounds very much like the one the Multiple Myeloma Research Foundation (MMRF) has used for many years. Since its founding in 1998 the MMRF has raised over $300 million for cancer research. But more importantly, the MMRF created a collaborative model whereby researchers who receive funding are encouraged to share their data and discoveries. The results speak for themselves: Ten new drugs have received FDA approval in record time, tripling the life expectancy of multiple myeloma patients.

The President's announcement came just a month after Congress passed an appropriation bill that increased funding for the National Institutes of Health by 6.6%, which includes a $264 million increase in funding for the National Cancer Institute. This was welcome news, especially since the budgets for cancer research had suffered some reductions during the previous few years. This appropriation not only restored those funds but increased them significantly.

President Obama asked Congress for $755 million for the Moonshot initiative for fiscal year 2017. Most of these funds will be allotted to the National Institutes of Health. The focus will be on enhanced early detection, prevention, vaccine development, immunotherapy, combination therapies, genomic analysis, enhanced data sharing, and pediatric cancer. An early effort will be to get more patients into clinical trials. Again, this parallels the efforts of the MMRF.

All of this is great news for those of us with multiple myeloma. We have seen great advances in the treatment of multiple myeloma in the past few years. I have attended many seminars in which I have heard researchers and clinicians say that we are close to a cure. Many new types of treatments are in the pipeline. The Moonshot initiative promises to speed up the quest for a cure by doubling the current rate of progress. Think of the progress that has been made in the last decade. Now double it. How can we not be excited?

Considering the advances that have been made in the past few years one might ask why we need to do more. Each year over 12,000 people in the U.S. die from multiple myeloma. For those patients, the new treatment options were not enough. The fact is that while most of us may benefit from the new drugs, many will not. We must do more for them. Even those of us who will benefit from recent advances may eventually run out of options. In the absence of a cure, myeloma survivors stay alive only by taking powerful maintenance drugs that have significant side effects that impact our quality of life.

> **Considering the advances that have been made in the past few years one might ask why we need to do more. Each year over 12,000 people in the U.S. die from multiple myeloma.**

As myeloma patients and caregivers, it is important for us to put pressure on our Congressmen and Senators to support this initiative and make sure that it is properly funded in the future. But we can do more. Research is expensive and government funding for cancer research needs to be supplemented with private funds from organizations such as the MMRF. That's where we can do our part. Right now, the MMRF needs funding to support new clinical trials that hold the promise of extending the lives of those of us who have multiple myeloma and may provide options for patients who have become refractory to current drugs. Researchers are currently investigating new classes of drugs, and new treatment options that have great potential, such as turning on the immune system to fight cancer. None of this can continue without sufficient funding and we must do our part

Each year the MMRF's Team for Cures sponsors a 5K walk/run in at least 13 cities throughout the U.S. This is an enjoyable way to help the MMRF as it works to bring new drugs and treatments to us. Consider joining a team or forming one of your own. As individuals, our contributions may be small, but collectively we can do much. If you live close to one of these cities, consider joining or forming your own team. If you do not live near one of the walks, consider being a virtual walker. For more information go to http://www.themmrf.org/events/races-or-team-events/5K-run-walk/. The MMRF also sponsors several other events throughout the year the give patients and families the opportunity to make a contribution. These are explained on their website under the "MMRF Events" tab.

The International Myeloma Foundation also sponsors several fundraising events each year. In addition to providing patient support, advocacy, and numerous patient services, the IMF promotes results driven research that has made significant inroads towards finding a cure. For more information, go to https://www.myeloma.org/get-involved.

Life is good.

9. Have You Heard These?

Once people hear that you have cancer, they are ready to offer all sorts of advice. While they mean well, sometimes they say things that really aren't all that helpful. Here are a few comments that I've heard that still make me smile.

> Here are a few comments that I've heard that still make me smile.

I know someone who has the same disease. He's run into all sorts of problems and he's not doing well at all.

Yes, there are complications and side effects. And the treatment doesn't always go well. I know that. I don't need to be reminded of it and I don't need to hear about all the awful things someone else has experienced. I need to think positive. I need hope and one good way for me to find hope is to hear about those patients who are doing well. I'd much rather hear some success stories.

My cousin's friend had a bone marrow transplant 20 years ago. You should talk to her.

It's always good to talk to someone who's been there, but if you do talk to another patient, make sure it's someone who has had the procedure recently or has kept up-to-date with what is being done now. There have been many advances in the past few years and what was done even five years ago, is now ancient history. If you do want to talk to someone, I would suggest finding a resource such as the Dana-Farber Cancer Institute's One-to-One program that matches newly diagnosed patients with those who have been there. The people who volunteer in these programs are trained to support newly diagnosed patients and stay abreast of changes in the field. It's a much better option than talking to the friend of a friend.

Now I bet you wish you had used sunscreen.

How many times have you had to explain that it's myeloma, not melanoma? And then they look at you as though you don't know what you're talking about. Even so, it's not a bad idea to use the sunscreen.

Boy, you really look good. I can't get over how great you look.

So how am I supposed to look? Should I look sick? Did you expect that I wouldn't have any hair or that I would have lost weight? Whenever someone tells me that I look good, I thank them, but then emphasize how well I feel. I think it's important for us to let people know that we can live normal lives despite having an incurable cancer. I always stress that how I feel is more important than how I look.

Is that a bad kind of cancer?

Is there a good one? I know that some cancers are worse than others and there are certainly many that are worse than multiple myeloma. However, I haven't yet found a good one.

Oh well, you have to die of something. Who knows, you could get hit by a bus tomorrow.

Yep, that's reassuring. But, I'll make sure I look both ways before I cross the street.

A stem cell transplant can't be all that bad. I met a guy yesterday who had one a week ago, and he was out on the golf course.

Hmmm, I think there's a little bit of misinformation there. He either had some other kind of procedure or he had a transplant a lot longer than a week ago. Or, maybe he was just ignoring his doctor's orders.

Did you ever think of taking supplements or trying alternative therapies? I've read a lot on the internet about people who have been cured of cancer by doing this.

No thanks. I'll stick to medical science if you don't mind.

I know just how you feel.

I appreciate the sentiment and the kind thought behind it, but unless you've had radiation, months of chemotherapy, and a stem cell transplant, then you probably don't know how I feel. Even Deb, who never left my side during all my treatment, acknowledges that she could never understand how I felt. And, by the same token, I could never understand how she felt watching it all. You truly can't understand until you've been through it.

Well, if I were you, I'd . . .

Well, you're not me. Again, the advice may be well-meaning, but it is probably not relevant.

God doesn't give you more than you can handle.

In that case, I wish I couldn't handle much. We are often the recipients of religious comments and advice. While I certainly appreciate someone telling me that they did something for me that was appropriate to their religious beliefs, such as praying or lighting a candle, I don't need to be told that I should do something of a religious nature. My religious beliefs are personal, and I do what's consistent with them. What's right for someone else may not be right for me and may even be inconsistent with my own religious beliefs and practices.

Everything is going to be all right.

Again, people mean well with this comment and are trying to be reassuring. For most of us it is an innocuous comment. But for patients and their caregivers who are dealing with the final stages of disease, this can be a very unsettling statement. If you don't know that everything is going to be o.k., then it's best not to say it.

Everything happens for a reason.

That may be true, but it still isn't reassuring. I will admit that many good things have happened to me since my diagnosis (which I address in a future chapter), but even that doesn't make me feel better about having cancer.

Life is good.

10. Preventing Multiple Myeloma

In the past decade, the research into finding better treatments, and even a cure, for multiple myeloma has been nothing less than dramatic. During that time 10 new drugs to treat myeloma have received FDA approval and the life expectancy of myeloma patients has tripled. I am, however, struck by the fact that not much research has gone into how multiple myeloma can be prevented to begin with. Perhaps this is because a definitive cause of myeloma has not yet been identified.

Two recent studies do suggest that many cancers, and deaths from cancers, can be prevented by lifestyle changes.

The first study, published in the journal JAMA INTERNAL MEDICINE, suggests that exercise can lower the risk of getting 13 types of cancers, including multiple myeloma. Although many studies have shown that people who are physically active are less prone to developing certain types of cancers, this is the first that I am aware of that specifically references multiple myeloma.

The study's authors found that moderate to vigorous exercise significantly lessened the chance of developing the 13 cancers. Further, the risk decreased for those who exercised more. Those who spent the most time exercising had as much as a 20% reduced risk of developing the 13 cancers studied. The researchers do not fully understand how physical activity reduces cancer risk, but the important fact for us is that the study strongly suggests that exercise can reduce an individual's risk of getting multiple myeloma.

In the second study, published in JAMA ONCOLOGY, the researchers conclude that half of all cancer deaths and the development of 40-60% of new cancers could be prevented by lifestyle changes. We are all aware of the benefits of not smoking and drinking only in moderation, but the study's authors also conclude that maintaining an appropriate weight and exercising play an important role in preventing cancer.

While the second article did not specifically mention multiple myeloma, the two studies combined provide a strong indication that exercise and nutrition play an important role in the prevention of cancers, including myeloma.

So, what does this mean for those of us who already have multiple myeloma? Could adopting a healthy lifestyle, that includes good nutrition and regular exercise, help us in fighting our disease? Could it help to prevent or postpone a relapse? I know of no studies that answer those questions in the affirmative, but I do know a couple of oncologists who would answer them with an emphatic "Yes!" Our doctors are doing all they can to improve our prognosis and extend our lives. We must do our part and exercise and nutrition are factors that are in our control.

> **Could adopting a healthy lifestyle, that includes good nutrition and regular exercise, help us in fighting our disease?**

Equally as important, adopting a healthy lifestyle may help prevent us from getting other cancers. Cancer is one of those things where more isn't better. And of course, a healthy lifestyle helps to prevent other maladies, such as heart disease.

So, does this motivate you to want to do better with your diet and exercise? Help is available. The Livestrong Foundation has partnered with YMCAs across the country to offer free or low-cost fitness programs for cancer patients. These programs are run by trainers who understand the needs of cancer patients. Many cancer centers also have exercise physiologists who can help you develop an exercise routine suited to your needs. Likewise, most cancer centers have nutritionists who can help with diet planning.

Although I never had an unhealthy lifestyle, exercise and diet were two areas where I could improve. I'm far from perfect, but since being diagnosed with multiple myeloma I have tried to do better in this regard. Even before I came across the two recent studies, my oncologists stressed the importance of the role of diet and exercise as part of my overall treatment plan.

As far as my diet is concerned, I must give Deb all the credit. She works hard to plan healthy meals and makes sure that I stay away from junk food. When shopping, she doesn't buy snack foods like cookies or chips. As she says, "If I buy them, you'll eat them." She's right. When I want a snack, I grab something like fruit, yogurt, or nuts. I do have one vice—ice cream.

As far as exercise is concerned, I'm not one to go to a gym. Instead, I bought a treadmill and an elliptical machine and try to spend an hour exercising 4 to 5 days a week. Admittedly, it is the longest hour of the day. Do I enjoy it? No, but life is good, so I'll continue. I get through it by visualizing cancer cells being crushed underneath my feet.

In the better weather, we stay active by going for walks and gardening. During the winter, it is harder to be active, but here in the northeast Mother Nature provides us with the opportunity by giving us our fair share of snow to shovel.

Have these lifestyle changes helped? I really don't know for sure, but I certainly think so. At this writing, I've been in remission for almost nine years and I feel that diet and exercise have been factors. So, I'll continue to eat right, and several days a week I'll make the trek downstairs to work out on those infernal machines.

Life is good.

Sources:

Moore, S., et al. *Association of Leisure-time Physical Activity with Risk of 26 Types of Cancer in 1.44 Million Adults.* JAMA INTERNAL MEDICINE. http://archinte.jamanetwork.com/article.aspx?articleid=2521826&version=meter+at+2&module=meter-Links&pgtype=Blogs&contentId=&mediaId=%25%25ADID%25%25&referrer=http%3A%2F%2Fwww.nytimes.com%2Fsection%2Fhealth&priority=true&action=click&contentCollection=meter-links-click (May 16, 2016).

Song, M. & Giovannucci, E. *Preventable Incidence and Mortality of Carcinoma Associated with Lifestyle Factors Among White Adults in the United States.* JAMA ONCOLOGY. http://oncology.jamanetwork.com/article.aspx?articleid=2522371 (May 19, 2016).

11. The Bucket List

I recently read an online article about people in their later years who were asked what they wished they had done more of in their lives. One item that was on the top of the list was traveling more. This answer resonated with me because Deb and I enjoy traveling and have been very fortunate that we have been able to do so.

I think most of us have bucket lists of things we would like to do. It may include trips we would like to take, tasks we want to finish, old friends we want to reconnect with, or even new things we would like to learn. For many people, new experiences are on the top of their bucket list. They want to travel, experience other cultures, meet new people, learn something new. When talking about this I often hear people say, "Someday I'm going to …"

> **I often hear people say, "Someday I'm going to …" For cancer patients, someday is today.**

For cancer patients, someday is today. Even those of us who are in long-term remissions know that our time may be limited. Yes, it's true that most people walking around today don't know how much time they have. But cancer patients, even those like myself who have reason to be optimistic, live with the knowledge that we have a disease that puts some limits on our life expectancies.

So, like most people, Deb and I have bucket lists of things we want to do and places we want to go. But we have also learned to not put the bucket list on hold for someday. Like everyone else, our budget is not unlimited, so we have to set priorities. As soon as we check off one item on our bucket list, we add at least one more.

So, what's on your bucket list? Is there some place that you'd really like to visit? What have you been meaning to do but haven't gotten to yet? Are there things that you'd like to have, but you really don't want to spend the money? What are your priorities? It's important to set your priorities and then work out a plan to reach them.

In my opinion, the first thing that should be on the bucket list of anyone newly diagnosed with cancer is to make sure that all your affairs are in order. This is not something we like to talk about, but knowing that your financial, legal, and other matters are in order gives you peace of mind. Once you have taken care of this, you can begin doing the fun things.

For us, travel is always on the top of our bucket list. Even though we've been lucky enough to travel extensively, there are still more places we would like to visit and many places we would like to return to. We have set travel as a priority and do without other things so that we can travel. Are there places you would like to go? Have you dreamed of visiting Paris in the spring? Perhaps you'd like to make an excursion to the place where you grew up. Now's as good a time as any to make those plans.

For other people a new purchase may be a priority. Are you a sports fan or movie buff who has always wanted a big screen TV to better experience your passion? Well, don't feel guilty. Get it now while you can enjoy it. I am always reminded of our former neighbor who, as he approached 80, decided to buy a new car. He told me he didn't want anything fancy or with a lot of options. He set off to buy that car but came back with a red sports car that was loaded. He saw it on the dealership lot, fell in love with it, and bought it. He has enjoyed that car greatly for several years. More power to him!

Most people enjoy spending time with friends and family. There never seems to be enough time to do that. Often, we take our friends and family for granted, assuming that they will always be there. Now is as good a time as any to make this a priority. It's also a good time to reconnect with old friends and relatives you haven't seen in a long time. Have you ever wondered what happened to some old friends from high school or college? Why not look them up and send them an email or call them.

Don't wait until it's too late. Take some time to sit down with your bucket list, set your priorities, and start working on it. Someday is here.

Life is good. Live it.

12. The Silver Lining

We have all heard the proverb "Every dark cloud has a silver lining." The meaning behind this proverb is that something good can come from misfortune. I think all of us will agree that being diagnosed with multiple myeloma was a dark cloud. It may have even been the darkest cloud in our lives. Does the dark cloud of myeloma have a silver lining? The answer for me is an emphatic "Yes!" In fact, my dark cloud has many silver linings. Many good things have happened to me, not only since my diagnosis, but because I have multiple myeloma. I believe that these things have enriched my life and have made me a better person.

> Many good things have happened to me, not only since my diagnosis, but because I have multiple myeloma.

Deb and I have always had a circle of very good, close friends. Since my diagnosis, we have added to that circle. We have met some wonderful people who are part of the Multiple Myeloma Patient and Caregiver Education and Discussion Group at the Dana-Farber Cancer Institute (DFCI) where I was treated. Perhaps because we all have a very common bond, many of the participants in this group have become quite close. We have also met many delightful, caring people through our volunteer work at DFCI and our association with the MMRF. Again, perhaps what makes these people special to us is that we share a collective mission. The friends we have made through these connections are among our most cherished, and we wouldn't trade them for anything. Yes, our new good friends are certainly a silver lining.

When Deb and I retired, we knew we were too young for the rocking chairs. We planned to take a little time off and then look for some volunteer opportunities. Before we had the chance to even think about what kind of volunteer work might interest us, I was hit with the cancer diagnosis. That put life on hold for over a year, but once I had recovered we both knew exactly what we wanted to do. We wanted to do something to help pay back for all that had been done for us and to help other cancer patients. We have become involved in several activities. One of the most rewarding is that we are peer coaches with the One-to-One program at DFCI where we provide support to newly diagnosed myeloma patients and their caregivers. We also participate in the MMRF's Team for Cures 5K Walk/Run in Boston every year. Walking with others to raise funds for a cure is inspiring. We volunteer for many other activities to support DFCI, the Jimmy Fund, and the MMRF. All of this makes our lives much richer. Yes, the various volunteer opportunities that have been dropped in our laps are more silver linings.

"Take the time to stop and smell the roses." "Live for today." "Enjoy every day to its fullest." "Don't sweat the little things." We have all heard these clichés. Since being diagnosed with multiple myeloma these sayings have taken on new meaning for me. My overall outlook on life has changed for the better. Now, I take the time to appreciate the little things in life. Most importantly, I have come to realize what's important in life. I appreciate every day and enjoy every moment. Yes, my greater enjoyment of life is another silver lining.

I no longer get upset over little annoying things. When you have been through what I have been through, those minor annoyances become very insignificant. For example, several months ago my car was hit in a parking lot. Prior to my cancer diagnosis this might have upset me. But, it was no big deal. The car could be fixed. Yes, the fact that I no longer get stressed out by trivial challenges is a silver lining.

Although I took all the required science courses in high school and college, I really don't have much of a science background. I was always more interested in history and the humanities. During the past few years I have substantially increased my medical knowledge. I am far from being an expert, but I find this new knowledge fascinating. Having multiple myeloma has opened a whole new area of learning for me. As we all know it is important to engage in life-long learning and keep our brains active. Yes, another silver lining has been the opportunity to explore a subject matter that I never knew much about.

These are just a few examples of positive things that have happened to me because I have multiple myeloma. Although I really would prefer not to have cancer, I also would not ever want to have my friends, volunteer opportunities, and current outlook on life taken away from me. I am very grateful for all of them. I think my new perspective in understanding the true meaning of life is the ultimate silver lining.

Life is good.

13. Why Not Me?

When first diagnosed with cancer, many patients ask themselves, "Why me?" When I asked myself that question, the answer I gave myself was, "Why not me?" Cancer touches so many people. I honestly couldn't come up with a reason why it should not hit me. Sure, for the most part I took care of myself, tried to live right, and didn't have any particularly bad health habits. Even so, there was no reason why I couldn't get cancer just like everyone else.

This past year has been one of reflection for me. I have once again been asking "Why not me?" but in a different context. Recently, several fellow cancer patients I have gotten to know quite well have relapsed and too many have passed away. Most of them were diagnosed after I was. I have been very fortunate that my myeloma remains in remission. Nevertheless, their experiences have made me think, and I have to wonder, "Why not me?" Why have others relapsed and I haven't?

Despite all the advances that have been made in the treatment of multiple myeloma in the past decade, it is still considered to be an incurable disease. The odds are that we can all expect a relapse at some point. We don't like to think about it, but the fear is always present. We may suppress it, but it is still there.

When I go in for my periodic check-ups, a bit of anxiety creeps in. Will this be the time the lab results aren't what I want them to be? Deb and I wait anxiously for the electrophoresis tests to come back and it is usually an emotional moment when we see the report that tells us that all is well. We usually look at each other with tears in our eyes and say, "We're so lucky."

When I hear of fellow patients who have relapsed I get that sinking feeling, "Will I be the next one?" "When will my time come?" I have no reason to feel that I will be next or even that a relapse is in the near future. After all, I have been firmly in remission for almost

> **When I hear of fellow patients who have relapsed I get that sinking feeling, "Will I be the next one?" "When will my time come?"**

nine years and lab results show no signs of myeloma. However, as I have seen in others, that can change unexpectedly. There are times when I wake up at night and the fear grips me. I wonder if the fact that I have gone this far without a relapse only means that one is right around the corner.

Does this bit of fear make me a pessimist? No. I think it makes me a realist. I know what the statistics say, and I recognize that a relapse at some point is possible, even likely. But, despite the fear that occasionally intrudes, I remain a very positive, optimistic person who feels in my gut that I am not about to relapse any time soon. In fact, I am optimistic that I have beaten this disease.

Am I conflicted? I suppose I am to a degree. Even though I remain very optimistic, I must admit that I have moments when the fear of a relapse that is always present somewhere in the back of my mind rears its ugly head. I keep that fear suppressed by reminding myself of the many reasons why I don't expect to become a statistic. I focus on those positive test results that have been coming in since I first heard those words, "You're in remission." I remind myself how lucky I have been and how fortunate I continue to be.

So, why not me? I don't have an answer. Hence, although I live with the knowledge that my time may come some day, I try not to dwell on it. Instead, I endeavor to live for today and just enjoy life. That sounds like a cliché, but for those of us with an illness that is considered to be incurable, it is not. With the knowledge that things can change, Deb and I don't put off doing those things that we really want to do. We don't go around saying, "Someday we'd like to ..." We recognize that someday is today and we need to do the things we really want to now. On the other hand, because we are optimistic that I'll be around for quite a while longer, we also make long-term plans for the things we'd like to do next year, and the year after that, and the year after that ...

Life is good. Embrace it. Every single minute of it.

14. Tips for the Newly Diagnosed

For most people, getting a cancer diagnosis comes as a shock. I was blindsided with my own diagnosis because I really did not feel that I was high risk for cancer. Quite frankly, with my family history I was more concerned about other diseases. A cancer diagnosis is devastating. When you are given the diagnosis, your first reaction is "How much time do I have?" Soon you begin to think of the treatment and wonder how awful it will be.

I have been diagnosed with cancer twice. The first time was the multiple myeloma diagnosis. The second one was prostate cancer. From my experiences, I have a few tips for newly diagnosed myeloma patients and their caregivers.

> **From my experiences, I have a few tips for newly diagnosed myeloma patients and their caregivers.**

Don't waste your time being angry. Feeling angry when you are first diagnosed is natural, but it won't change things. Instead, focus on enjoying every minute of every day. When I get up in the morning, if it's a nice, sunny day I say, "Wow, what a great day to be alive." If it's a cold, miserable, rainy day I say, "Wow, what a great day to be alive." I find it easier to remain optimistic by not allowing anger to be part of my life.

Take things one step at a time. When I was first diagnosed, my oncologist told me that we were going to take things one step at a time. Depending on the characteristics of your disease, there may be several steps in your treatment. It's o.k. to want to know what's next, but it's important to concentrate on what you are doing in the present. Don't get too far ahead of yourself.

The treatment won't be easy, but you can do it. There will be some tough days. Depending on your treatment you may experience side effects such as nausea, fatigue, or gastrointestinal problems. There will be quite a few days where you just don't feel well. But these days will soon be over and better days are ahead.

Stay focused. Concentrate on getting better and always keep the end result in mind. Don't let the little things distract you. It helps to visualize. When I was hooked up to the IV getting my chemo I closed my eyes and visualized all those cancer cells meeting their demise. It made me feel better.

Talk about it. It might be hard, but it is important to talk about what you are going through and how you feel. This is also a very hard time for family and close friends and it helps them if you share with them. They will never truly understand what you are going through, but they want to. Don't shut them out. Include them.

Tell your doctors and nurses everything, even if you don't think it's important or significant. They are not being polite when they ask, "How are you feeling?" They really need to know. This is no time to be a hero. Remember, when you tell your doctors exactly how you are feeling, you are not complaining. You are giving your medical team valuable information. They cannot fix it if you don't tell them what's wrong. So, let them know if you are nauseous, if you are in pain, if you are having trouble sleeping, or anything else that is not right or normal.

Accept the help you need. Many people will offer to help. If you need help, take them up on the offer. But, you must be very clear about what you need. By the same token, be clear about what is not helpful.

Above all else, be positive! I like to say that my motto and my blood type are the same – Be positive and B positive. Positive thinking goes a long way in helping to beat this disease. It may be hard some days, but it is important to stay focused and to stay positive.

Ask questions and get as much information as you can. When you meet with your medical team ask for clarification of anything you don't understand. If you still don't understand, say so. Ask your doctor where you can get more information. Be careful using the internet. Many internet sources are not reliable. The International Myeloma Foundation and the Multiple Myeloma Research Foundation are great sources of information. The *Myeloma Beacon* is another good one.

Write your questions down ahead of time and bring them to your appointment. You will likely have many questions. When you are at the appointment it's easy to forget one or two of them. To make sure you ask all the questions you have, write them down, bring them with you, and refer to them during the appointment.

Do what your doctors tell you to do. They know what they are doing. They don't put restrictions on you just to be mean. There is a reason for all the rules. Follow them.

If you want a second opinion, get one. It's never a bad idea to get a second or even a third opinion. Don't be afraid of hurting your doctor's feelings by asking for another opinion. Chances are, your doctor will also appreciate getting the opinion of another expert.

Don't ever give up. We have many reasons for hope. Although multiple myeloma is incurable, many advances in its treatment have been made in the past few years. Many more are in the pipeline and a cure may be just around the corner.

Life is good.

15. Questions to Ask Your Oncologist

A diagnosis of multiple myeloma can be overwhelming. For many people, the first time they ever heard of the disease may have been when they received the diagnosis. To better understand the disease, how it will affect you, and your prognosis, it is important to ask your doctor many questions. The problem is, that most of us, when first diagnosed don't know what to ask. If you have recently been diagnosed, here are a few questions you might ask your doctor.

> **If you have recently been diagnosed, here are a few questions you might ask your doctor.**

Tests and Lab Results

Over the course of your treatment you will be monitored very closely. As part of that process your oncologist will order many diagnostic tests. While the results of these tests give your doctor important information, you should also pay attention to them so that you can ask questions about changes.

What do all these lab results mean? How do I interpret them?

Which lab tests are most important to me? Which ones are specific to myeloma?

How often will these tests be done?

How will the results be reported to me?

Diagnosis and Treatment

Today there are multiple treatment options available. While your oncologist knows best which option is most likely to give you the results you want, it is important for you to understand all options and why a specific treatment plan has been developed for you.

What stage multiple myeloma do I have and what does it mean for treatment?

Do I have any molecular defects or genetic mutations that make my disease difficult to treat?

Are my kidneys or bones affected?

What can I do to prepare for treatment?

What are the available treatment options?

What treatment option do you think is best for me and why?

How soon should we start treatment?

Are there any clinical trials that might be open for me?

Would a clinical trial be better for me than standard treatment?

How will we know that the treatment is working?

Medications

Today many medications are available to treat multiple myeloma. Most patients are prescribed a cocktail of two, three, or even four drugs. It is important for patients, and their caregivers, to know as much as possible about these powerful drugs.

Why are you recommending these medications?

What are the most important things I need to know about my medications?

Will any of these medications interact with other medications or supplements I am taking?

Should my medications be taken with or without food?

When should I take my medications?

What should I do if I miss a dose?

Side Effects

Unfortunately, all treatments have side effects or unintended consequences. Most of these side effects can be tolerated or managed. They are simply the price we must pay to regain our health. Even so, some side effects can be serious and may affect how you are treated. It is important for you to understand all side effects and what should be done when you experience them.

What kind of side effects will I likely experience?

What can be done to mitigate side effects?

What side effects should be reported to a medical professional immediately?

If I experience serious side effects when your office is not open, who should I call?

Will there be long-term side effects that I will have to live with?

Lifestyle Changes

When you are diagnosed with multiple myeloma your life will change. That does not mean that life will not be good, it's just that it will be different. How good life will be may well depend on how you are able to adjust to your "new normal." You will be better able to make that adjustment if you are prepared for the changes.

What restrictions will I have as far as daily activities are concerned, i.e. what can I do and what can't I do?

Do I have any dietary restrictions?

How will my treatment affect my ability to participate in physical activities?

Will I need to make any other lifestyle changes?

How can I avoid infections?

Support

We all have different needs and different resources, but all of us will, at one time or another, need support during this journey. The good news is that support is available in several forms, such as individual counseling, support groups, and online forums. It's important to find out what's available and determine what will help you.

What is available for support? How do I access it?

Are there support resources for my family?

Financial Concerns

Multiple myeloma medications and treatment protocols can be expensive. It is important for you to understand what those costs are and how much of the cost you will have to shoulder yourself. If you need it, it is also critical for you to know what kind of financial assistance is available.

What will my insurance cover and what, if any, will I have for out-of-pocket costs?

If my insurance company refuses to cover certain aspects of my treatment, what options do I have?

If I can't manage the out-of-pocket costs, where can I go for financial help?

Follow-up Treatment

Since multiple myeloma is incurable, treatment never ends. Even after the major portions of our treatment are over, we will always need follow-up care and periodic tests for a relapse. Your medical team will give you a follow-up plan and it is important for you to understand what is required.

How often will tests be run to see if I have relapsed or need further treatment?

What tests will be given?

Who will coordinate my follow-up care?

What symptoms or changes should I watch out for?

What steps can I take to stay healthy?

When I see other doctors, what do they need to know about my condition?

If possible, it might be helpful to send your questions to your oncologist prior to your appointment. This will give the doctor time to think about them and prepare more informative answers. If you don't understand the answers you get, ask for clarification. Your diagnosis and treatment are much too important for you to not have a full understanding of the whole situation.

It's also a good idea to bring someone with you to the appointment. I have always found that two sets of ears are better than one. Deb very often picks up on things the doctor said that I missed completely. After each of my appointments we spend time discussing what was said to make sure that we both have a clear understanding.

Life is good.

16. Is it Chemo Brain or Am I Just Getting Old?

Most of us who have been through cancer treatments have experienced degrees of cognitive impairment commonly known as chemo brain. In addition to being in a general fog, we have had problems with memory, concentration, and being able to pay attention. Although chemo brain can be very frustrating, it becomes a fact of life and is just one of the things you must deal with as part of your new normal.

Although chemo brain has been the focus of recent research it is still not clear what causes it. As with many afflictions, it is probably caused by several factors working together. A cancer diagnosis is accompanied by much stress and anxiety and this can certainly affect a patient's cognitive functioning. Some cancers can also cause chemical or physical changes to your body that can interfere with your memory and overall ability to think. Finally, cancer treatments, and the complications that arise from them, can be the culprits.

> **Although chemo brain has been the focus of recent research it is still not clear what causes it.**

The degree and duration of chemo brain varies from one patient to the next and the kind of treatment you have had. In some patients, the effects of chemo brain necessitate a referral to a neurologist for diagnosis and possible treatment. However, the good news for most of us is that our overall cognitive functioning improves after we have finished our cancer treatment. Although it does get better, many of us find that we still have some remnants of chemo brain years later. Or is it that we're just getting older?

Throughout my career, I have done a fair amount of professional writing. When I retired, I planned to concentrate on a few projects that I had not gotten to while I was working. However, after I was diagnosed with multiple myeloma, I discovered that I just couldn't write anymore. I simply was unable to concentrate on what I was doing. I would start a paragraph and forget where I was going with it. It took me hours to write a few paragraphs that I should have been able to complete in a few minutes. The words just would not flow. It was so frustrating that I stopped writing altogether.

Even reading was a challenge. I couldn't concentrate well enough to follow a story line in a novel. Although I was going through the motions of reading, I'd find that I often had no idea what I had read in the previous few minutes.

Eventually, after I had recovered from my stem cell transplant, things got better. Although I still suffered from fatigue, my ability to concentrate got better. It wasn't as good as it once was, but it improved to the point that I could again enjoy reading a good book or sit down at my computer and write something coherent, as I hope I am doing now.

I still experience some cognitive problems. I find that I cannot multitask as well as I once could. I often get distracted and forget what I'm doing. Just the other day I went down two flights of stairs to get a screwdriver and a couple of screws. I got distracted and went back upstairs without them. On my second trip down, I got the screws but forgot the screwdriver. I finally got it right on my third trip. Maybe chemo brain is nature's way of getting us to exercise more.

One morning as Deb and I were having coffee we started to talk about the essays we were writing. I told her that I had started a new one but couldn't for the life of me remember what it was about. After a few minutes, I remembered, "Oh yeah, it's about chemo brain."

I have found that chemo brain provides a convenient excuse for those times when I really was just not paying attention. Like those times when I'm not listening to what someone else is saying and am later caught having not paid attention. In response to "But I just told you that," I can blame it on chemo brain.

I'm finding, however, that the chemo brain excuse doesn't always work. When I try to blame my forgetfulness on chemo brain, Deb reminds me that I am getting older. Unfortunately, she may be right. When I look in the mirror I do see more grey hairs than I used to.

Regardless of whether our cognitive difficulties are due to chemo brain or aging, we can do something about it. First, if you feel that it is a serious problem and is interfering with your quality of life, it is important to discuss it with your doctor. A consult with a neurologist may be in order.

If, however, your difficulties with cognition fall more in the category of a minor annoyance, brain exercises may help. In the same way that it is important to stay physically active, it is important to stay mentally active.

It is vital to always challenge our brains. Thinking and memory exercises are helpful. I enjoy trying to answer trivia questions or doing number puzzles. Some people benefit from crossword puzzles. I am constantly challenging myself to learn something new. It may not be something that I will use, but I feel that it is vital to learn for the sake of learning. The important thing is to just keep our brains working.

Life is good.

17. The Importance of Clinical Trials

Clinical trials are important in helping researchers develop new multiple myeloma treatments and better understand how the disease operates. Clinical trials have been instrumental in the development and approval of the drugs that are available to treat myeloma today. In fact, before any new drugs or procedures will be approved by the Food and Drug Administration for the treatment of cancers, or any disease, researchers must demonstrate that they are safe and effective in the treatment of a disease. This is accomplished by gathering data in clinical trials. Clinical trials remain a critical element in the search for a cure for multiple myeloma. The more people who enroll in clinical trials, the faster we will reach that goal.

There are also advantages for patients who enroll in clinical trials. These patients can be among the first to receive the newest and most promising treatments. They also receive very close monitoring of their disease. For patients who have relapsed or become refractory to current treatments, a clinical trial may offer renewed hope.

When many of us think of clinical trials, we think of the model where one group gets an experimental treatment, and another gets a placebo, or sugar pill. Clinical trials in multiple myeloma do not work that way. Patients in clinical trials receive either the experimental therapy or one of the current state-of-the-art treatments.

In deciding whether a clinical trial is right for you, you should keep in mind that the experimental treatments may be better than or at least equal to current standard treatment options. On the other hand, there is always the chance that the experimental treatment may not be as effective as current options. Also, since these treatments are still in the experimental stage, they may have unexpected side effects. Then again, many new treatments have fewer side effects than the current medications. Each of these factors needs to be weighed by any patient considering a clinical trial.

> In deciding whether a clinical trial is right for you, you should keep in mind that the experimental treatments may be better than or at least equal to current standard treatment options.

Your oncologist can help you evaluate the benefits and the risks of participating in a clinical trial.

It's easy to appreciate why some patients may be reluctant to enroll in a clinical trial. Understandably, many would prefer a known treatment option rather than take the risk for something that may, or may not, be effective. However, when considering a clinical trial, you should know that you will receive close monitoring during the trial, and if the experimental treatment does not seem to be working for you, or the side effects are particularly troublesome, you can always withdraw from it and go back to a standard treatment option.

There are three types, or levels of clinical trials, known as phases. In *Phase I* trials the safety and dosage of the drug is determined and information about how the drug is absorbed and acts in the body is gathered. *Phase II* trials assess the drug's effectiveness and safety. Finally, in *Phase III* trials, researchers compare effectiveness and safety of the experimental drug with standard treatments.

Perhaps one of the most compelling reasons for participating in a clinical trial is for the opportunity to help advance medical science. Your participation can help researchers gain important medical knowledge and improve patient treatment and care. In other words, by participating in a clinical trial, you provide a benefit to future patients by supporting the process that will bring them more, and better options. In this way, you will touch many lives.

The decision on whether to participate in a clinical trial is an important one. It is also very personal. You should discuss all options with your medical team. You need to fully recognize the risks, as well as the benefits, of your participation. Further, make sure you know and understand your responsibilities

You also need to understand the costs of participating in a clinical trial. There are no costs for the patient for the medications and tests that are conducted as part of clinical trials and your health insurance should cover other medically-necessary costs. However, there could be some incidental costs, such as transportation and lodging if you don't live near the site where the trials are conducted. Your participation also may require more of your time than would be required if you elected an established treatment option.

So, if you have the chance to participate in a clinical trial, give it some thought. Talk to your doctor about it. Weigh the pros and cons and decide what is best for you.

I, personally, have never had the opportunity to participate in a clinical trial. If, in the future, the opportunity presents itself, I think I would jump at the chance. The most significant criteria for me would be the prospect of being able to contribute to medical science and the ultimate quest for a cure. After all, the successful treatment that I received came about because someone else was willing to participate in clinical trials. Even so, I would take a close look at all options before deciding which one is right for me.

The Multiple Myeloma Research Foundation has an excellent tool to help you locate clinical trials. To find out more about clinical trials and to access this tool, go to https://www.themmrf.org/living-with-multiple-myeloma/clinical-trials-finder. Two other comprehensive and reliable places to search for clinical trials are the National Cancer Institute at https://www.cancer.gov/about-cancer/treatment/clinical-trials/search and the U.S. National Library of Medicine at https://clinicaltrials.gov/.

Life is good.

18. Taking Care of Yourself

As I'm sure all multiple myeloma patients are aware, having this disease puts us at risk for developing many other health issues. For example, because our immune systems are compromised, we are more susceptible to bacterial and viral infections. During periods when our immune systems are the most suppressed, most of us take antibiotic and antiviral medications prophylactically. Even so, we must always be on our guard to avoid infections.

As patients, it is easy for us to become so focused on our multiple myeloma that we neglect other aspects of our health. As we get older that can be a serious mistake because we are just as vulnerable to other ailments as everyone else, if not more so. Having multiple myeloma doesn't make us immune to other illnesses, or even other cancers.

It is incumbent on us to pay close attention to our general health. We have a much better chance of overall survival if we focus on all our health needs. Just as important, our overall quality of life will be better if we stay healthy. Here are a few basic things all of us should pay attention to.

> **It is incumbent on us to pay close attention to our general health. We have a much better chance of overall survival if we focus on all our health needs.**

Vaccinations. Most of us have had childhood vaccinations. The effect of those vaccinations can be wiped out by cancer treatment, especially a stem cell transplant. It is important to be re-vaccinated and to make sure you get all necessary boosters, especially considering recent outbreaks of diseases such as measles. At least once a year Deb and I ask my oncologist to review my vaccinations to make sure that all are up to date. And of course, the annual flu shot is practically mandatory.

Annual physical. Even though myeloma patients see oncologists on a very regular schedule, and get a multitude of blood tests, it is still important to make an annual appointment with our primary care physicians to have annual physicals. My myeloma was diagnosed early because of the diligence of my primary care physician – something for which I will be forever grateful. Several years later, a routine physical also led to an early diagnosis of prostate cancer. I now see many specialists, but I make sure that I have an appointment with my primary care doctor at least twice a year. I bring my latest lab reports from my oncologist to those appointments and we go over them together. He then orders tests and screenings that he feels I should have that were not included in the oncologist's workup.

In addition to monitoring my cholesterol, during my annual physical, my doctor checks my heart, cardiovascular, and pulmonary systems. He monitors my blood pressure, evaluates my blood sugar, and screens me for other maladies. Given my family history of heart disease and diabetes, this is important. My primary care physician is the gatekeeper who monitors my overall health and makes recommendations for me to see other specialists as needed. This is one appointment I will never put off.

Annual skin check. Most of us grew up in an era when we spent time baking in the sun without benefit of sunscreen. Unfortunately, for many of us, the sins of our youth have caught up to us. I also visit a dermatologist at least twice a year. I have had many precancerous moles removed from various parts of my body. These check-ups make sure that anything suspicious is taken care of before it becomes a problem. Two types of cancer are enough – I don't need a third.

Gastrointestinal evaluations. Regular colonoscopies are important for everyone. How often you have one depends on your family history as well as your own prior colonoscopy results. One of my doctors tells me that one every ten years is fine for me, but another recommends one every five years. As much as I dread them, I prefer to err on the sooner rather than later side. Our myeloma treatments regimens can also cause many other gastrointestinal disturbances, most temporary, but some permanent. Even years after my treatment ended, I have some lingering digestive problems that may, or may not, have been caused by the chemo. Regardless, I now have regular visits to a gastroenterologist.

Dental care. Regular cleanings and dental check-ups have become routine for most of us. This is especially important for those of us who are taking bisphosphonates. A rare, but nasty, side effect of some bisphosphonates is osteonecrosis of the jaw (ONJ). Proper dental hygiene can help to prevent ONJ.

Optometric exams. Face it, we're all getting older. I find that these days I can't read anything without my reading glasses. Holding printed material out at arm's length doesn't help anymore. Annual optometric exams are a way of life for most people over the age of 50. Cancer treatments can cause problems such as dry eye and cataracts. Shortly after I finished my chemo, my eye doctor told me that I had cataracts. These may be due to the chemo or they may just be part of the aging process. Either way, my optometrist keeps a close eye on them (no pun intended).

Various other specialists. Depending on our own individual circumstances, we may need to periodically visit other specialists, such as urologists, podiatrists, rheumatologists, etc. If we need them, it is just as important to see these specialists according to their recommended schedules.

The bottom line is that in addition to seeing our oncologists on a regular basis, most of us have an army of other medical professionals that we see throughout the years. This means that we always seem to have an upcoming appointment with someone. It can be tedious, but it's a small price to pay for staying alive, being healthy, and enjoying life.

Life is good. And it's better when we stay healthy.

The Patient

19. Taking Care of Your Caregiver

November has been designated as National Family Caregivers Month. Although most caregivers are related to us, we often receive care and support from non-family members such as friends and colleagues. Regardless, November is a time for us to reflect on the important role our caregivers play in our overall treatment.

In my opinion, our caregivers have a much harder job than we as patients do. They are on duty 24/7 and don't get any paid holidays or vacations. It can be very stressful watching a loved one go through treatment. Caregivers are often told that to be effective they must take care of themselves first. I often joke with Deb about taking care of herself, saying, "If anything happens to you, who will take care of me?" But there is a lot of truth to that.

Our caregivers are very important to us. They are a critical part of our overall health care team. Where would we be without them? I shudder to think how I ever would have gotten through this journey without Deb at my side. While it is true that they must take care of themselves so that they can better care for us, there is much that we can do to make sure that they remain healthy. In other words, we need to take care of our caregivers.

> **Our caregivers are very important to us. They are a critical part of our overall health care team. Where would we be without them?**

Sometimes our caregivers are so focused on us, they forget their own health. They may put off making appointments for themselves for routine care such as an annual physical. They may even ignore ailments that should be looked at. Because they accompany us to our numerous appointments, our caregivers may not take the time to schedule appointments for themselves. We need to give them gentle reminders, and even insist if necessary, so that they will go to doctors when they need to.

I recall a time when my father was caring for my mother who had Alzheimer's disease. When I noticed that he was neglecting his own health and talked to him about it, his response was "I don't care what happens to me." I had to remind him that my mother would be lost without him, and that it was important for him to keep up with his own health care. When he thought about it, he agreed that I was right.

Our caregivers' social lives also suffer because we may be limited in what we can do. Particularly after a stem cell transplant, when we are isolated from the world, our social activities are significantly curtailed. However, that doesn't mean that our caregivers must also be isolated. We need to encourage them to take time out to visit with friends, go out to lunch, and do some of the things they would like to do.

Let's face it, after a stem cell transplant, taking care of us is no picnic. There is so much we can't do ourselves. When I was at my worst, Deb had to not only do the household tasks she usually handled, but she also had to take on everything I did. On top of that she had the responsibility of meeting my health care needs. Add to that the worry of living with someone who was seriously ill. If that isn't a recipe for stress, I don't know what is.

What can we do to relieve some of that stress? Well, we can start by not doing anything to add to it. In this respect, I think it's important to make sure that all our legal and financial affairs are in order so that our caregivers don't have to worry about that. But we can also make sure that our caregivers get proper rest, eat well, and get some exercise. We should encourage our caregivers to accept some help from others when they need it. We need to let them know that it's o.k. for friends and other family members to give them a break now and then.

I remember the first time Deb went out with some friends when I was in treatment. She was reluctant to leave me, and I think she went only because she didn't want me to feel badly if she declined their invitation. She did, however, ask Ed, a neighbor and good friend, to come over to keep me company. While I didn't think that I needed a "babysitter," I realized that she would feel much better knowing that someone was with me. To give her peace of mind so that she could enjoy herself more, I consented to having Ed come over. Ed and I had a nice visit and Deb had a much-needed break.

We should be diligent in watching for signs that our caregivers are experiencing some burnout. If we think they are, then we should encourage them to take some steps to mitigate it. One thing we can do to help prevent burnout is to encourage them to spend some quality time doing the things they enjoy. If they are not already part of one, we might encourage them to join a support group for caregivers. Helping them to maintain a sense of humor can also be beneficial.

And finally, but probably most importantly, we need to let them know how much we appreciate everything they do.

Life is good. But it's good because we have such good caregivers.

The Patient

20. The Gift of Time

Deb and I recently attended a funeral where the priest's homily was about how precious time is and how we don't always recognize that fact. He began by asking, "How many of you got up today and thanked God that you were alive?" We looked at each other and silently acknowledged that we did, as we do every morning. In fact, I often say that when I get up on a nice, sunny day I look out the window and say, "Wow, what a great day to be alive." But then again, when I get up on a cold, snowy, miserable day, I look out the window and say, "Wow, what a great day to be alive."

The priest also relayed a conversation he had with his brother where they talked about the fact that because they were now part of the so-called older generation, they needed to do the things they really wanted to do. They recognized that even though they were healthy, they had more days behind them than ahead of them. The point the priest was making in his message was that none of us really know how much time we have, so we need to use it wisely. In his experience, most people take time for granted and don't think about it. Consequently, they realize too late that they have not done some of the things they really wanted to do in their lives.

On our way home Deb and I discussed the homily and what it meant to us. While we agree with the priest that most people do take time for granted (as we once did), in our experience most cancer patients and their caregivers do not. Going through any kind of serious illness, such as cancer, makes you understand how lucky you are to be alive and makes you appreciate life more. But it also makes you very aware of how finite life is. We are well-aware that every day is a gift and that we need to live life to its fullest.

> **Going through any kind of serious illness, such as cancer, makes you understand how lucky you are to be alive and makes you appreciate life more. But it also makes you very aware of how finite life is.**

We were recently featured in an article in a special edition of *Health Monitor* magazine entitled "Living with Multiple Myeloma." The editors gave the article the headline: "My someday is today." That headline came from a statement I made to the article's author that Deb and I live each day to its fullest and that we don't put off doing the things we really want to do. We often hear people say, "Someday I'm going to do such and such." But for us, and everyone surviving cancer, someday is today because we don't know what tomorrow will bring. We don't put anything off for a special occasion because, for us, just being alive is a special occasion.

As I stated in an earlier essay, Deb and I had just retired when I was diagnosed with multiple myeloma. The ensuing treatment put our retirement plans on hold for well over a year. Once I was well enough to resume normal activities, we decided that we really needed to make the most of each day. We very much realized that we were given the precious gift of time. But we also realized that the gift was not ours to keep forever. Although we don't know when it is, that gift has an expiration date. Those of us who have multiple myeloma live with the reality that our cancer is incurable and that it can come back at any time.

Having that gift of time meant that we could travel, do things together, and enjoy life. But it also meant that we had time to do some good. We had been given a very special gift, one that is not given to everyone. We knew we needed to make good use of it by giving back. For us, that meant doing some volunteering in the cancer community. Although our motivation for volunteering is to give back, we have found that our volunteer activities have enriched our lives and made them more meaningful. It may be a cliché, but we truly get more than we give.

The bottom line is that we are having the time of our lives. And that just makes us want to savor the gift of time all that much more.

The gift of time is the most precious gift you will ever get. You may only get it once. So, use it wisely.

Life is good.

21. Beware of Charlatans Selling Snake Oil

If, at the beginning of my multiple myeloma journey, my oncologist gave me the choice between undergoing radiation, chemotherapy, and a stem cell transplant or taking a pill that would not cause any side effects, which do you think I would have chosen? When faced with a cancer diagnosis we would all like to find that magic pill or elixir that will cure our disease without all the side effects of traditional treatments. Unfortunately, such a magic cure does not exist.

We are bombarded in the media by advertisements for all sorts of supplements that purport to cure or relieve a myriad of ailments. We hear about "natural" pills that will help us lose weight without dieting or exercise, remedies that will relieve us of many of the ailments that come about as part of the aging process, and various potions that will turn us into almost superhuman beings.

Unfortunately, cancer patients can be barraged by false and exaggerated claims regarding alternative therapies that supposedly will cure their disease. Recently, while searching for books about multiple myeloma in an internet bookstore, I found several books by authors who claimed to have been cured by such alternatives. I have also seen many posts in online patient forums by people who swear by certain dietary supplements.

> **Unfortunately, cancer patients can be barraged by false and exaggerated claims regarding alternative therapies that supposedly will cure their disease.**

Well-meaning friends, and even other patients, may tell you about all kinds of supplements, foods, or other treatments that they believe will cure you. How many of us have been told by an acquaintance that they read an article about an extract from the root of an exotic tree that was proven to cure all types of cancer? My usual response to such claims is, "Show me the science." The fact is, if these claims were supported by legitimate, scientific research, our doctors would already be using these treatments.

The federal Food and Drug Administration (FDA) has an ongoing effort to protect consumers from health fraud. As part of that effort the FDA regularly issues warning letters to companies that make claims to prevent, treat, or cure various diseases without evidence to support those claims. These companies take advantage of cancer patients by playing on their fears and their desperation to find a cure. Making such unsubstantiated claims violates federal law.

A quick perusal of the agency's website shows that in 2017 alone it warned 18 companies to stop making claims that their products could treat or prevent cancer. In the past decade the FDA has issued over 90 warning letters to companies marketing products they fraudulently claimed treated cancer. These companies made claims such as "combats tumor and cancer cells" and "makes cancer cells commit suicide without killing other cells." The sheer number of warning letters that have been issued shows that we must be suspicious of the claims made for any supplement or alternative therapy.

Not only are the claims made about the products in question unproven, but according to the FDA, many of these products may even contain harmful ingredients and can adversely interact with other medications. Again, because very little, if any, legitimate research has been done on these products, not only have they not been proven to be effective, they also haven't been shown to be safe.

You also must beware of miracle treatments that claim to be backed up by research. Research can be faked, or results misinterpreted to "prove" the claims. Just because a product claims to be backed up by proven research, doesn't mean it is so. One trick often used by supplement companies is to make an unproven or outright false claim in large print and then put a disclaimer about the product in small print. The old adage to always read the fine print is good advice. Some advertisements are accompanied by testimonials from "patients" who claims to have been cured. Very simply, such claims can't always be trusted.

Many people believe that if something is natural it can't hurt you, but this is not always the case. Many natural products can be harmful. First, they can be dangerous if you reject standard treatments that have a good chance of working in favor of alternatives that don't. Second, many supplements are known to counteract, interfere with, or adversely interact with prescription medications and can be dangerous when taken in conjunction with other therapies. Supplements also can be dangerous when used to excess and many supplements have undesirable side effects.

That is not to say that all supplements are bad. Some have been shown to be beneficial in mitigating the side effects of treatments. When I was discharged from the hospital after my stem cell transplant, I was given several medications along with some vitamins and supplements prescribed by my doctor.

I am not saying that you should not take any supplements, but you should take them only with the consent of your doctor. Your doctor knows the science and can help you differentiate between the legitimate claims and the scams. So, before you take anything, make sure you discuss it with your doctor.

Life is good.

Part III: The Caregiver

1. In Sickness and in Health

On that beautiful day in October, filled with all the excitement life had to offer, I didn't realize how important those words would become. Caught up in the wonderment of our wedding day, the magnitude of those words did not resonate with me until 2008 when my husband was diagnosed with multiple myeloma.

Until you have experienced the overwhelming shock a diagnosis of cancer brings to an otherwise healthy person, I am not sure that you can truly understand the impact. Many people facing any of life's challenges ask, "But why us?" I never asked that question. After all, cancer touches nearly everyone, so why should we be any different?

If it had been me with the cancer I could have dealt with it more easily. Finding out that the person I loved more than life itself had cancer was the biggest challenge of my life. I vividly remember silently wishing the situation were reversed.

Being a strong believer in the fact that life holds no guarantees I accepted the fact that my husband was the patient and I was, what is known in the cancer world as "the caregiver." I remember hearing the word *caregiver* for the first time and thinking of it as a bit odd. I knew, as any grade school child can tell you, that the word caregiver is a compound word meaning one who gives care. But, in this whole new world of mine, what did that actually mean?

When my husband's medical team used the word, they made it sound almost like a vocation, much like a teacher or a firefighter. I felt as if I was holding the most important position in the world and I hadn't even applied for the job. I began asking myself if there were qualifications. Obviously, I didn't need a resume, but what exactly was my role? Was I qualified?

I learned quickly that the role of a caregiver was not defined. There was no road map, no directions, no GPS that would take me from point A to point B, and

> **I learned quickly that the role of a caregiver was not defined. There was no road map, no directions, no GPS that would take me from point A to point B, and certainly no one to tell me how long that journey would take.**

certainly no one to tell me how long that journey would take. Instead I needed to figure out what my role in this journey would be. I needed to look at our relationship and contemplate what was most important for us. I needed to learn how best to be supportive without being controlling and how to be understanding and compassionate without being overly sympathetic. Finding the balance has not always been easy, and like any new job, I have stumbled along the way and hopefully learned from my mistakes.

I set out thinking that maybe in writing this chapter I could help provide tips for navigating the caregiver's role, but as I think about conversations I have had with other people in similar situations, I realize that the role of caregiver is as varied as the diagnosis of cancer itself. There is no one size fits all. Each patient and each caregiver is uniquely different and consequently their needs are different.

Caregivers do have one significant thing in common that binds us tightly together: We continue to believe in the future, confident that a cure is not far away. So, my advice - after seven years on the job - is to take one day at a time, do not become overwhelmed with what may come next, and simply ...

Don't stop believing.

2. Multiple Myeloma...What's That?

Someone you love and care about has just been diagnosed with multiple myeloma. You know the diagnosis is not good, but you really don't know anything about it. Questions swirl in your mind.

What exactly is it?
How did he or she get it?
What is the treatment and prognosis?
How can I help?

In this chapter I am trying to answer these critical questions as simply as possible. There will be plenty of time to learn more about multiple myeloma later. Right now, you need to have these key questions answered.

First, what is multiple myeloma? As explained in the first part of this book, multiple myeloma is a blood cancer that develops in the bone marrow. Bone marrow is the soft spongy tissue found in the center of many bones where blood cells are produced. In myeloma, plasma cells, which are normal antibody-producing cells, transform into cancerous myeloma cells. Myeloma cells produce large quantities of abnormal antibodies. These cancer cells crowd out and inhibit the production of normal blood cells. The complete definition of myeloma is much more complicated than I have stated here, but for initial purposes it is probably all you need to know for now.

To address the next question of how did he/she get it? The answer to date has not been clearly defined. According to the MMRF's website, research suggests possible associations with a decline in the immune system, exposure to certain chemicals, exposure to radiation and certain occupational hazards. For example, the likelihood of multiple myeloma is higher than average among people in agricultural occupations, petroleum workers, workers in leather industries, and cosmetologists. Exposure to herbicides, insecticides, petroleum products, heavy metals, plastics, and various dusts including asbestos also appear to be risk factors for the disease. However, there are no strong connections with these associations and in most cases multiple myeloma develops in individuals who have no known risk factors. Multiple myeloma may be the result of several factors acting together.

The treatment and prognosis questions are complicated. The diversity of the disease makes this question dependent on many factors. The prognosis of multiple myeloma is usually based on the existence of different signs, symptoms, and circumstances. Certain tests results provide important information and help decide when treatment should begin and aid in monitoring the disease. Multiple myeloma's prognosis as well as survival rates have improved significantly due to myeloma research. For more detailed information regarding this question, I urge you to go to MMRF's web page entitled "About Multiple Myeloma," at https://www.themmrf.org/multiple-myeloma/what-is-multiple-myeloma/. On that page there is more information as well as a number you can call to speak directly to a nurse specialist who can help answer your specific questions.

Lastly, answering the question of what you can do to help is pretty basic. Simply be there. Be there to listen and support your loved one in any capacity necessary. Depending on your relationship with the patient, be that spouse, partner, relative or friend, let them be your guide. Your role is crucial to their prognosis.

> **Answering the question of what you can do to help is pretty basic. Simply be there.**

Being diagnosed with cancer is difficult for any individual, but having someone who can provide comfort, strength and hope during this challenging time is monumental.

Don't stop believing.

3. Just Breathe...

In agreeing to chronicle our journey through Allan's diagnosis and treatment of multiple myeloma, I am reminded that our story isn't much different than thousands of others diagnosed with multiple myeloma. In fact, in many ways our story, although challenging, has been and fortunately remains very optimistic. We consider ourselves the luckiest people in the world.

As I reflect on Allan's regimen of treatment, namely radiation, chemotherapy, and ultimately a stem cell transplant, I realize how much multiple myeloma has and continues to play a role in what has shaped our lives for the last nine years.

Each treatment has brought its own host of side effects such as fatigue, gastrointestinal issues, neuropathy and infections. While these are minor considering the big picture, watching a loved one deal with these issues can be difficult. While you understand the necessity for each treatment and are truly grateful that those treatments are available, as a caregiver, sometimes you do feel a sense of helplessness.

In speaking to other caregivers, I hear many concerns regarding the stress of caring for a loved one with a cancer diagnosis. That stress can be due to the overall anxiety related to the diagnosis itself, trying to deal with financial issues, or providing comfort and reassurance to children. For a caregiver, that stress can manifest itself in the form of loss of appetite, difficulty sleeping, or an inability to concentrate.

> **In speaking to other caregivers, I hear many concerns regarding the stress of caring for a loved one with a cancer diagnosis.**

In terms of dealing with that stress, I am reminded of something I was once told by another caregiver. After boarding a flight, prior to takeoff, the flight attendant recounts all the safety procedures for the aircraft. You are reminded that you need to place the oxygen mask on yourself before assisting others, including small children.

We as caregivers need to follow this important rule as well. We need to remember that we cannot effectively do our job if we do not first care for ourselves. It may seem at times that you have no extra time to care for yourself, but it is imperative that you allow yourself permission to take that time. Whether that simply means having dinner with a friend or going for a bike ride - do something nice for yourself.

So just breathe, inhale that oxygen and know that you are a valuable part of a very special team.

Don't stop believing.

4. Thank you!

Allan and I have always tried to keep up with what the researchers are doing in the multiple myeloma field. We often attend patient seminars sponsored by organizations such as the Multiple Myeloma Research Foundation. In 2015 we attended one such patient summit hosted by the MMRF in sponsorship with various pharmaceutical companies including Bristol-Myers Squibb, Celgene, Genentech, Janssen, Onyx, and Takeda Millennium.

The program featured many highly-acclaimed researchers in the field of multiple myeloma, including Drs. Kenneth Anderson and Paul Richardson from the Dana-Farber Cancer Institute in Boston who co-chaired this extraordinary program. The summit, which the MMRF offers each year in various locations across the U.S., is open to all multiple myeloma patients and their caregivers free of charge.

The seminar began with an overview of multiple myeloma, simply entitled *Multiple Myeloma 101: Diagnosis, Prognosis and Risk* presented by Dr. Nikhil Munshi from Dana-Farber. That session was followed by an update pertaining to first line treatment for newly diagnosed patients, given by Dr. Paul Richardson. The next topic addressed was by Dr. Amrita Krishna from the City of Hope in Los Angeles entitled *Hematopoietic Cell Transplantation for Multiple Myeloma*, in which she outlined the entire process of a stem cell transplant, including the medical rationale for having a transplant.

Following her presentation, we were treated to lunch, giving us the opportunity to interact with other patients and caregivers. I always find it interesting to speak with others regarding their diagnosis and progress. Through exchanges like these, we have met some incredibly inspirational people.

The afternoon's session began with a very comprehensive presentation by Dr. Jacob Laubach of Dana-Farber detailing the management of multiple myeloma as well as treatment for relapsed/refractory disease. He was followed by Dr. G. David Roodman from Indiana University who provided us with insights into the changing paradigm of managing multiple myeloma. The final speaker was Dr.

Kenneth Anderson. He focused on preclinical and early phase clinical trials, and probably what is most important to all myeloma patients, promising new treatments.

It is difficult to accurately describe just how much critical information was presented by each doctor. Their expertly delivered presentations were highly detailed, yet still understandable from a layperson's perspective. As I reflect on all that I took away from this summit, the most important part of the day was the underlying message of hope that was evidenced by each presenter: Hope for a future in which a cure will soon be found. Such a great feeling!

> **As I reflect on all that I took away from this summit, the most important part of the day was the underlining message of hope that was evidenced by each presenter: Hope for a future in which a cure will soon be found.**

We are truly fortunate that the MMRF and other organizations provide the opportunity for all of us to attend these events. If you have not attended one in the past, I urge you to participate in the future. Not only does it allow us to become more informed and better educated patients, but it gives us something to believe in.

Thank you to all who make these events possible.

Don't stop believing.

5. The Tough Question

Several years ago, Allan and I were fortunate enough to be part of a specialized training program to become mentors in a program called One-to-One at the Dana-Farber Cancer Institute in Boston. In that capacity, we are matched with newly-diagnosed multiple myeloma patients. Our role is to help them navigate through the complex issues surrounding diagnosis and treatment. The goal of the program is to provide support, understanding, and - most importantly - hope.

In speaking with other caregivers of newly-diagnosed myeloma patients, I am faced with a myriad of questions regarding patient care and expectations. Usually the questions can be easily answered. They range from dealing with healthcare insurance to dietary restrictions after a stem cell transplant.

But there is one question that I continue to struggle with, and I am unable to provide a suitable answer. I almost dread the inevitable fact that it will come up in conversation. The question simply is, "When will the worry go away?" I distinctly remember the first time I was asked the question. The sadness in the eyes of the woman who asked it, not only brought tears to my eyes, but made me realize that I never actually thought about it. The "worry" had simply become part of the journey - much like the diagnosis itself. It went to bed with me at night and awoke with me each morning. As I pondered the woman's question, I really didn't know how to answer.

> But there is one question that I continue to struggle with, and I am unable to provide a suitable answer…. "When will the worry go away?"

I knew that I wanted to say something that would provide comfort and reassurance, but I also wanted to make sure that my answer was truthful. I spent a great deal of time reflecting on how to answer such a critical question.

While I would never presume to speak for all caregivers I can say that for me, with time the worry no longer plays a major role in our lives, but remains, nonetheless. I think that it sits deep in the recesses of every patient and caregiver's mind. Most often it goes unspoken.

So, I am challenged with answering the ultimate question, "When does the worry go away?"

I really don't know. I wish I had a better answer. I can say - as we all know so well - that life presents many challenges and many worries, but somehow, we manage. We continue to move forward taking one day at a time. I have learned to focus on the fact that each day is precious. No day slips by unnoticed. They are all gifts.

At the beginning of Allan's diagnosis, I adopted three simple yet very powerful words - "Don't Stop Believing." Those are the words that I live by; those are the words that guide me, knowing that each day we are closer to a cure. Those are the words that I share with all those who ask, "When does the worry go away?"

Don't stop believing.

6. November is National Family Caregiver Month

Each year the President issues a proclamation designating November as National Family Caregiver Month. That proclamation recognizes that each day courageous individuals step forward to help care for family members in need. Their quiet acts of selflessness tell stories of love and devotion.

In light of that proclamation I would like to pay tribute to those caregivers. Since November is also a month in which we traditionally give thanks, I would like to thank all caregivers for everything they do.

> **Since November is also a month in which we traditionally give thanks, I would like to thank all caregivers for everything they do.**

As you know from our previous essays, Allan and I spent our careers in education. At this time of year, it was customary at our schools for teachers to ask their students to create what we refer to as an acrostic poem. It is a poem in which you begin with a word and create thoughts, ideas, or sentences beginning with each letter of that word. The first letter of each line in the poem then spells out the word, similar to a simple acronym. In November, we would ask our students to create their own acrostic, reflecting on those things for which they were thankful.

This month I have chosen to make an attempt at creating an acrostic poem for caregivers using the simple, but very powerful, word **THANKS**. It is my way of acknowledging all that caregivers do for their loved ones.

> **T**he month of November is designated as Caregiver Month.
> **H**undreds of thousands join their ranks each year.
> **A**ttempting to provide comfort to those they love most.
> **N**ever giving up hope.
> **K**nowing the challenges that lie ahead.
> **S**taying strong.

It is with thanks that Allan and I extend gratitude to those who are such an important part of a very special team. Your tireless efforts and deep compassion in caring for others are not only acknowledged but are counted among those things for which we are most grateful. Without you the journey for those facing multiple myeloma would be far more challenging.

Don't stop believing.

7. Diet and Nutrition

I am sure that I have already discouraged some people from reading this essay because of the title *Diet and Nutrition*. We have all heard time and time again the importance of eating healthy and getting enough exercise. We are bombarded with it daily on the news. You can hardly pick up a magazine that doesn't have an article related to the benefits of regular exercise and nutritious eating. With this constant assault, many people become overwhelmed and confused. Unfortunately, some people stop listening.

When Allan was diagnosed with multiple myeloma the importance of diet and exercise became even more critical to us. There wasn't anything we could do about the cancer, but we could do something to ensure that he was as strong and healthy as possible prior to the treatments he would undergo. It was something that we could control. Initially, our world had been turned upside down and it seemed like our destiny was being dictated by the cancer. So, knowing that there was indeed something that we could do, for me, was empowering.

> **When Allan was diagnosed with multiple myeloma the importance of diet and exercise became even more critical to us.**

Allan and I have always tried to be aware of what we eat and the importance of being active. We regularly attend seminars regarding diet and exercise. They make us reflect on the importance of staying active and eating well. We are far from perfect in either area so that gentle reminder that we are doing the right thing is helpful in keeping us on track. I am hoping that the information in this chapter, while not new, causes you to reflect as well.

I came across some tips for eating healthy put out by the American Cancer Society. The tips are simple and easy to follow.

- Read food labels to become more aware of portion sizes and calories. Be aware that "low-fat" or "non-fat" does not necessarily mean "low-calorie."

- Eat smaller portions when eating high-calorie foods.

- Choose vegetables, whole fruit, legumes such as peas and beans, and other low-calorie foods instead of calorie-dense foods such as French fries, potato and other chips, ice cream, donuts, and other sweets.

- Limit your intake of sugar-sweetened beverages such as soft drinks, sports drinks, and fruit-flavored drinks.

- When you eat away from home, be especially mindful to choose food low in calories, fat, and added sugar, and avoid eating large portion sizes.

As far as exercise is concerned, there are numerous statistics as to what you should be doing each day. The guidelines for some can be challenging, especially for those patients undergoing the rigors of treatment. Seeing those statistics may cause some to get discouraged if they aren't close to meeting the recommendations. For that reason, I love Nancy Campbell's philosophy. Nancy is the exercise physiologist at the Dana-Farber Cancer Institute in Boston. She says that you should simply try to do more than you did yesterday. If you could only do a 10-minute walk today, congratulate yourself and try to do just a little bit more tomorrow.

Think of simple ways to increase your daily amount of activity. Parking your car in a spot further from your destination is one we all know, but Nancy suggests using the rest room on a different floor from the one you work on if that is a possibility. Be creative, I bet you can think of several ways to increase your daily amount of activity. The important message is just keep moving. Research consistently shows that physical activity also reduces stress. The benefits are endless.

In an essay in the next section we highlight four new drugs approved by the FDA in 2015 for the treatment of multiple myeloma. The advancements in just the last few years have been unprecedented. We live in incredible times. As I reflect on all that is being done in terms of research and treatment, I feel that there is something that we can do as well. Our part is to stay as strong as possible. Eating well and being active is our part of the equation.

While the diagnosis of multiple myeloma was certainly not a choice, we do have a choice in how we respond to it.

Don't stop believing.

8. Ask Not...

In other chapters Allan and I have written a great deal of information regarding the incredible developments made in the field of multiple myeloma. We are humbled by the advancements made by dedicated researchers in the last decade. These treatments are providing hope to many myeloma patients. In view of all this encouraging news, we should pause and remember that, although the arsenal of medications for fighting multiple myeloma is large, the cure remains elusive. Even with all the breakthroughs that have been made, for some myeloma patients it still is not enough. They are in a race against time.

For that reason, the funds needed to support research are critical. I believe as patients and caregivers we need to accept the responsibility of doing our part to make sure that the dollars are there to support that research. We cannot simply stand by and wait. We must become more involved in helping to find that cure.

> I believe as patients and caregivers we need to accept the responsibility of doing our part to make sure that the dollars are there to support that research.

I am reminded of a time, more than fifty years ago when President Kennedy called our nation to action in his famous inauguration speech when he said:

> *Ask not what your country can do for you, ask what you can do for your country.*

If we reflect on those words and apply that concept of a call to action to multiple myeloma, then maybe we should:

> *Ask not what the doctors and researchers can do for us, but ask what we can do for the doctors and researchers.*

The answer is simple—more funding. The solution is much more challenging-where will that funding come from?

In 2016 President Obama proposed an initiative calling for increased funding for cancer. It was anticipated that the new funding would not all come from the government but would come from private sources as well. One private source is the MMRF. Each year the MMRF sponsors various events to raise funds and awareness. One event that is particularly special to Allan and me, is the Team for Cures 5K Walk/Run that is held in a variety of locations throughout the year. Funds raised from this event have helped to:

nearly triple patient survival
deliver ten new treatments in a decade
launch over 60 new clinical trials

In 2010 Allan and I formed *Team Snug Harbor*. In 2017, collectively, the Boston event raised more than $700,000. We are truly proud of all those who made that event so successful.

Below is a link that lists the dates and locations of the MMRF's Team for Cures events. As patients and caregivers, we are in a race that we must win. We encourage you to support an event in your area. Click the link for more information.

https://www.themmrf.org/events/races-or-team-events/

Be a part of the team that cures cancer once and for all.

Don't stop believing.

9. Is the Glass Half Full or Half Empty?

As I have mentioned in other chapters, our volunteer work affords Allan and me the opportunity to meet many new patients and caregivers. We are frequently asked how we have been able to remain so optimistic considering the diagnosis. For those of you who have followed our journey, you know how incredibly lucky we have been, but I think the main reason we are so optimistic is that we subscribe to the philosophy that the "glass is half full"

When Allan was diagnosed with multiple myeloma, although we were shocked and apprehensive, we remained very hopeful. In essence we saw the glass as half full. In no way do we consider ourselves exceptional individuals, so I began to wonder what shaped our view of the glass.

There have been several factors that have played an integral part in contributing to and sustaining our optimism. I am hoping that in sharing them it may help others in their journey.

First and foremost, we have complete confidence in the doctors and nurses who comprise our medical team. Collectively we make decisions, and once a decision has been made, we do not second guess it. We don't dwell on the what if's or the unknowns. We simply make the best decision based on the information we have at the time. Prior to making any decision regarding Allan's course of treatment, I always ask the doctors what they would do if they themselves were in our situation. That question has always been answered after considerable thought with true honesty.

Many people struggle with ultimately trusting the advice of their doctors and nurses, but in our experience, we have always found reassurance and support. If you do not establish a trusting bond with your medical team, the process of dealing with multiple myeloma is filled with anxiety and doubt. In my opinion, it is critical, from an emotional standpoint, to be able to confide in your medical team and trust their recommendations.

Second, we make every effort to educate ourselves concerning all aspects of multiple myeloma. There are countless seminars, webinars, and literature sponsored by both the MMRF as well as the International Myeloma Foundation that provide us with accurate information regarding current treatments. By keeping abreast of the current information, we can ask our medical team pertinent questions regarding Allan's care. Being an informed patient, gives us a feeling of having some control over the disease. That sense of control, coupled with all the new research being done in the field, adds to our sense of optimism.

Third, we continue to set goals. Short term, as well as long term, goals help us to normalize our lives and give us even more reason to look to the future. They can be something as simple as traveling to a new place, seeing the sights, and enjoying what the day has to offer. Or they can be long term like seeing our youngest niece graduate from college. The point is that we try to move forward, enjoying each day to its fullest.

Last, but certainly not least is our ability to find humor along the way. Truly, there is nothing comical about a diagnosis of multiple myeloma, but there are things that happen along the way that can be humorous and put a smile on your face. We look for those things and enjoy them together.

As I have stated elsewhere, being diagnosed with multiple myeloma was not our choice, but we do have a choice in how we perceive it. For us, we have chosen to see the glass half full. This view of the glass has given us strength, courage and the never-ending gift of hope.

> **As I have stated elsewhere, being diagnosed with multiple myeloma was not our choice, but we do have a choice in how we perceive it.**

Don't stop believing.

10. My Tom Brady

As a caregiver, I am often asked how we have coped with the challenges of Allan's multiple myeloma diagnosis. I think the best way I can describe what truly has helped us is that we work as a team. As I reflect back on the last nine years, our team has become more focused and ultimately stronger; much the same as all teams do when they play for multiple seasons. With time, you understand better each other's strengths and use them to their fullest capacity. While each of you clearly plays a different position on the team, you have the same ultimate goal...to win.

With the fall season, upon us and living in New England, I liken us to our New England Patriots. Allan being my Tom Brady and me being his Bill Belichick. Our discussions regarding what we need to do to win are of utmost importance. We look at all the options, evaluate the risks and decide on the best course of action. By continually working on improving the team's strength, both physically as well as emotionally, we remain focused on moving forward.

> **We look at all the options, evaluate the risks and decide on the best course of action.**

While I know that my position on the team is certainly important, I am very aware that I am not the one who is actually on the field taking all the hard hits. I am not the one who physically and emotionally endures what it is really like to have a cancer diagnosis.

My position instead, places me on the sidelines, watching and hoping that the strategies and decisions we have made together work. But in essence, I know that once my Tom Brady is on the field, there is little I can do. While I have the advantage of seeing the entire field, this vantage point poses my most difficult challenge. I can anticipate what will happen next, but there is little I can do to change the outcome. Like Bill, I have the option of calling a time out, but those time outs are limited and need to be used wisely. These are the times, as a coach or a caregiver, that are most difficult. So, I have learned to take deep breaths and put my faith in Allan as Bill has with Tom knowing that he needs to make some decisions on his own.

Each game, like each monthly blood draw is met with a degree of apprehension and anxiety. No matter how well prepared you may be, no matter how much you have trained, you don't know how things will turn out. Will we win this time? Will those monthly blood counts still be in check?

While the Patriots play each game in hopes that they will go to the playoffs and possibly on to win the Super Bowl, we too have similar hopes and aspirations. The difference being for us, the stakes are much higher. Will Allan continue to defy the odds? Will he remain in remission? When will a cure for multiple myeloma be found?

Like this year's football team, we don't have the answers to those questions, we just have to wait and see. Although waiting is challenging, we do know that for us, right now, we're fortunate to still be in the game.

Don't stop believing.

11. Just a Little More Time

In 2016 Allan and I had the opportunity to hear Vice President Joe Biden speak at the Edward M. Kennedy Institute in Boston. He spoke compassionately about his role in leading the Cancer Moonshot task force, whose mission is to dramatically accelerate efforts in preventing, diagnosing, and treating cancer. The essence of Biden's speech, or more accurately his personal plea, was "to change cancer as we know it" and move closer to a cure. Since President Obama appointed him to lead the task force, Biden has met with patients, caregivers, researchers, physicians, and other experts to better understand the challenges that impede the progress of moving toward finding a cure.

As you know the Vice President lost his son Beau in May of 2015 to brain cancer. In speaking of his son, he said that when he lost Beau he lost his soul. His voice quivered when he relayed the stories of countless, courageous patients pleading with their doctors to give them just a little more time. The thought of having to plead with a doctor for three more months, two more months, just a little more time to put your affairs in order and provide for your family is heart-wrenching.

> **The thought of having to plead with a doctor for three more months, two more months, just a little more time to put your affairs in order and provide for your family is heart-wrenching.**

As I sat and listened to his speech, I heard in his voice a deep commitment to move forward in finding a cure. I also heard what I have heard in the voices of others whose loved ones have succumbed to cancer. It is a voice filled with immeasurable loss — a loss so deep it can never be filled...an emptiness that even time cannot erase.

As the Vice President described Beau's plea for just a little more time, it made me pause, as well as we all should, to re-evaluate our priorities. The Cancer Moonshot Initiative should be placed at the top of our list. It is too late for Beau and many others, but it should not be too late for those facing a cancer diagnosis today.

It was back in 1971 that President Nixon first declared a war on cancer, a war that must be won. Although incredible progress has been made since that time, it is still not enough. The National Cancer Institute estimates that in the year 2016, in the United States alone, 1,685,210 new cases of cancer will be diagnosed, and 595,690 people will die from the disease.

Oftentimes, as a society we become complacent because an issue does not personally touch our lives. But the impact of this issue is so immense we cannot simply stand by; we need to take action and support the efforts of collaboration of information not only in accelerating awareness but in funding this important initiative.

As a patient or caregiver, I urge you to read our chapter in Part IV entitled *Cancer Moonshot—Progress and Promise*. In it we detail the initiative's findings as well as its hopes for the future. After reading this chapter, we hope that you will take the time to contact your local elected officials and impress upon them the priority of this issue. The Cancer Moonshot Initiative provides all of us with the never-ending gift of hope, but that hope diminishes when we don't act.

Someday may we live in a world devoid of cancer, where no one needs to plead for a little time.

Don't Stop Believing.

12. In the Blink of an Eye

Prior to Allan's multiple myeloma diagnosis, like so many other people we went through life in somewhat of a protective bubble. We never gave much thought to how quickly life can change direction.

Each day we hear many stories in which people's lives have been suddenly altered by an illness, or worse yet, a sudden unexpected death. We all empathize with each story, but until it directly affects our lives, I am not sure that we realize the exact impact of what it actually means to have your life change in a mere blink of an eye.

Allan's diagnosis of multiple myeloma in 2008 not only impacted our lives but changed us as well. It made us stop and pay attention to all the little things in life. It made us reassess our priorities. It gave a definitive meaning to the simple phrase, "All you need is your health."

As you know from our previous essays, Allan continues to do remarkably well. Except for a few bumps in the road along the way, we have been the lucky ones. Not a day goes by that I do not reflect on how fortunate we have been. We never buy lottery tickets, because in my mind we have already won.

Like so many things in life, with time comes complacency. That complacency was shaken recently when one of our friends who had been diagnosed with multiple myeloma four years earlier had a sudden relapse. The myeloma was not only back but it returned in a highly aggressive form.

In the last several months he has endured a rigorous treatment of both chemotherapy and radiation. As many of you know, those treatments come with significant side effects.

He has valiantly struggled and now is doing somewhat better, but it has not been without an immense amount of courage and determination.

His experience like that of so many other myeloma patients makes me reflect on how fragile life can be. How we really don't know what the future holds. After working for many years as an elementary school teacher I still find myself equating life's circumstances to characters in picture books. So, for me, myeloma is similar to living with a sleeping dragon. If you tiptoe quietly around him, maybe he will continue to sleep, but you always need to be mindful that at any time he can raise his ugly head.

What I find most incredible is how myeloma patients and their caregivers deal with such uncertainty. When our friend was asked how he stayed so focused and determined he simply said, "You play the hand you're dealt." May we all take strength in his courage and the courage of countless others facing similar challenges.

> **What I find most incredible is how myeloma patients and their caregivers deal with such uncertainty.**

During each day, no matter how busy Allan and I may be, we pause and remember that we must never take even the smallest of gifts in life for granted. Each day needs to be cherished. While setting long-term goals is admirable and necessary in many aspects of our lives, it is each individual day that really matters.

If this journey has taught us nothing else, it has taught us, what I consider the most valuable lesson of all: *Carpe diem* - "Seize the day" ... and trust no tomorrows!

Don't stop believing.

13. It's an Honor

Since Allan's diagnosis of multiple myeloma in 2008, we have made every effort to devote as much of our free time as possible to promoting awareness of the disease, raising funds for research and most importantly, volunteering in any capacity to help others face the challenges that come with a cancer diagnosis.

Allan, as you know, is being treated at The Dana-Farber Cancer Institute in Boston. Like many facilities, Dana-Farber has a group of devoted individuals called the Friends of Dana-Farber whose mission is to raise much-needed funds for research. The Friends have funded instrumental cancer research since 1976. In that time, they have raised more than 33 million dollars to not only promote promising research, but care and support programs across all treatment areas.

One such program sponsored by the Friends that Allan and I have become involved in is the distribution of gift bags to patients receiving infusions, as well as those waiting on the clinical floors for appointments. The gift bags are filled with personal care items such as lozenges, hand cream, lip balm, hand sanitizer and various other items that may be helpful to patients.

But this essay is not about what Allan and I do. In fact, it is not even about the gift bags. It's about the people we are privileged to meet when we deliver the bags. It's about their determination and resiliency to face whatever lies ahead. It's about their ability to accept their circumstances and continue to bravely face each day. Most of all, it is about their jubilation in one another's success stories.

As we deliver each bag, we let patients know that our gift is given with the hope that it will bring a little bright spot into what is a challenging point in their lives. Our small token is accepted with gratitude that manifests itself in the form of smiles, hugs, and oftentimes tears. It is at that point that so many people want to share their stories with us. They are stories that we know well. They are stories of

> Overwhelmingly, however, they are all stories of hope. Hope not only for themselves but hope for others.

challenges and victories. They are stories that make us rejoice and stories that make us pause. Overwhelmingly, however, they are all stories of hope. Hope not only for themselves but hope for others.

We receive much more than we give on bag delivery days. We have the privilege of experiencing that special bond that exists between patients. There is a comradery that is too difficult to put into words. I guess maybe because it is not something you can describe, it is something that you feel. It is a feeling of compassion and understanding that transcends all boundaries. Each time we deliver gift bags to patients we are in awe of their courage, their strength and their overwhelming concern for others.

For us, the delivering of bags is an honor. We consider ourselves truly fortunate to be able to surround ourselves with such inspiring people.

May they always possess the never-ending gift of hope.

Don't stop believing.

14. An Inspiration to Us All

All of you who follow our monthly posts on the MMRF's CoMMunity Gateway or who have been reading this book know that we consistently promote both awareness of multiple myeloma and the need for raising funds for research.

We have stressed the importance of funding that research, not only because it benefits myeloma patients, but because that research often leads to discoveries in other cancers as well. We have pointed out the accomplishments made by the MMRF and its mission to relentlessly pursue innovative means that accelerate the development of next-generation treatments to extend the lives of patients and lead to a cure. We do this to encourage people to participate in one of the Team for Cures events. It is anticipated that in 2018 the thirteen 5K Walk/Run events held throughout the country will generate over 3.7 million dollars for research.

As our team, along with 85 other teams, began to prepare for 2017 Boston race held on April 30th, we noticed a new team, organized by a very newly diagnosed patient. What caught our attention was the immediate support this team received from family and friends. On the day of the event, the team, Pinch's Punch Back, had 181 members and had raised close to $53,000. It is a true testament to what one family can do.

I guess what I found so inspiring about this team was not only the support that the Pinciaros received, but the fact that the diagnosis was so recent. Generally, newly diagnosed patients are just trying to comprehend the meaning of their diagnosis and are not even considering how in essence to pay back those who have gone before them in raising funds for today's current treatment.

> **Generally, newly diagnosed patients are just trying to comprehend the meaning of their diagnosis and are not even considering how in essence to pay back those who have gone before them in raising funds for today's current treatment.**

Through the help of the MMRF staff, Allan and I were able to contact the Pinciaros and ask them what it was that caused them to participate in the race at such a challenging point in their diagnosis. The answer they gave was heartfelt. To find out more about multiple myeloma, which affects over 30,000 new patients a year, they realized the importance of awareness.

The Pinciaros are like many families facing an unfamiliar disease. The overwhelming shock of being diagnosed with a type of cancer that most people have never heard of, is frightening. John Pinciaro had done everything right. He subscribed to a healthy diet and exercise plan. He had no underlying health issues and maintained a positive outlook on life. So, being diagnosed with multiple myeloma was in some ways inconceivable.

His story is not very dissimilar to many others, barring one very exceptional point. John and his family immediately realized that this was not only about him, this was about all those people facing the same diagnosis. This was about making people aware and raising necessary funds to further research.

In an effort to obtain as much information surrounding multiple myeloma as possible, Tiffany Pinciaro, John's daughter, came across the MMRF's website and the Team for Cures. During John's chemo treatments, the family organized a team of family and friends to participate in this year's race. Their take-charge mission is not unlike the mission Kathy Guisti began in 1998. They are people who see a need and immediately call to action the necessary resources to obtain that goal. They are people, who in the midst of a challenge, set high standards and with determination and courage press forward. They are people who set an example for us all. The Pinciaros are making a difference in the lives of many. A more admirable goal is difficult to find.

Allan and I consider ourselves fortunate to have met the Pinciaros. They left a lasting impression on us of what one family can do. We hope they inspire others, as they have inspired us, to continue to raise awareness and support the funds necessary to finding a cure.

I always end my essays with the words, "Don't stop believing" for I am convinced that one day that elusive cure will be found. Meeting John Pinciaro and his family, gives me a reason to continue to believe.

Don't stop believing.

15. Be Mindful

By the end of April, many myeloma patients and caregivers begin to relax about being cautious during cold and flu season, however according to the Center for Disease Control (CDC), Flu season can extend well into the month of May. Considering that myeloma patients' immune systems are compromised, continuing to be diligent about exposure to a variety of illnesses is extremely important. I thought it might be a helpful reminder to provide tips on keeping as healthy as possible during a time when many people because of the weather are in close contact with one another. It is noteworthy to point out that myeloma patients are about 15 times more likely to get an infection than people without myeloma.

> I thought it might be a helpful reminder this month to post tips on keeping as healthy as possible during a time when many people because of the weather are in close contact with one another.

Much of the information I have gathered comes directly from the CDC, which has an extensive website on staying healthy.

Tips for Staying Healthy

Frequent handwashing: Simply put, handwashing with soap removes germs. This helps prevent infections because people frequently touch their eyes, nose, and mouth without even realizing it. Germs from unwashed hands can be transferred to other objects, like handrails, table tops, or toys, and then transferred to another person's hands. Simple handwashing reduces diarrheal illness in people with weakened immune systems by 58% and reduces respiratory illnesses, like colds, in the general population by 16-21%.

Diet: The importance of drinking enough fluids and eating a well-balanced diet cannot be over emphasized. Staying hydrated and getting the proper nutrients by eating a diet high in fruits, vegetables and whole grains, and low in saturated fat is critical for keeping your immune system as strong as it can be.

Reducing Stress: This tip always makes me ponder the fact that it is much easier said than done, however, many studies have proven that decreasing your stress level can certainly affect your ability to ward off illness. Many people find it helpful to practice stress reduction techniques such as yoga and meditation. We personally find it helpful to surround ourselves with positive people. For us, people who appreciate the small things in life and try to focus on the things they can change rather than those things that they cannot help to keep us positive.

Rest: Get enough sleep each night. Sleep loss not only plays a role in whether we come down with a cold or flu, it also influences how we fight illnesses. If your immune system is already compromised your chance of contracting an illness is even greater. Allowing your body time to help repair itself through sleep is very important. Our immune system is designed to protect us from colds, flu and other illnesses, but when it is not functioning properly, it fails to do its job. The consequences can include more severe symptoms as well as a longer recovery period.

Exercise: The *Physical Activity Guidelines* recommend that adults get at least 150 minutes of moderate-intensity aerobic physical activity. Walking is a great way to get the physical activity needed to obtain health benefits. Walking does not require any special skills. It also does not require a gym membership or expensive equipment. If you can, try adding walking to your day.

Staying Away: Socializing with others, going places and doing things that you enjoy are all part of staying healthy, but staying away from people who may be sick is also very important. For us, the staying away tip proves to be the most challenging. There are so many situations related to work or family obligations where you simply have no idea who may be sick and avoiding them is impossible. If you are invited to a party, dinner with friends, or any social event in which you know some people have recently been contagious, you may want to rethink attending or at least be aware and practice good health habits. We have found our friends and family are very much aware of the limitations involved with having a compromised immune system and go out of their way to protect us.

I realize that these tips are not new to you, but if you are like me, sometimes you may become complacent and need a reminder to get back on the important track of keeping yourself healthy.

Don't stop believing.

16. Just Let Me Know

When hearing that someone has been diagnosed with cancer, we often respond with, "If there is anything you need, please let me know." While this comment is truly heartfelt, the problem is that many times cancer patients are just trying to comprehend the meaning of their diagnosis and cannot even begin to figure out what they may need.

In a discussion with other caregivers and patients who had been diagnosed several years ago, we talked about what it was that they remembered others had done for them in those first few critical weeks after being diagnosed. Of course, depending on the individual's circumstances, their responses were different. The needs of a parent dealing with the stresses of a young family are quite different from someone who may be living alone and has mobility issues. The point is, there is always some act of kindness, no matter how small it may be, that can provide comfort to a newly diagnosed patient.

> **The point is, there is always some act of kindness, no matter how small it may be, that can provide comfort to a newly diagnosed patient.**

In this essay, I thought it might be helpful to share some of the group's ideas for providing comfort and support to a newly diagnosed patient.

First and foremost is to respect someone's wishes for what will be helpful. Each patient deals with the diagnosis differently and those that offer their help need to understand that while they may not handle the situation in the same way, it is the cancer patient's decision to decide what is most beneficial for them. Once you have established the fact that the patient would appreciate help, you might like to consider some of the following suggestions.

For a parent with children an offer to provide transportation to and from their child's hockey practice, dance or flute lessons could be comforting. Taking their children to the library or possibly helping them with a special project that must be done for school was also mentioned. If a child's mom or dad cannot attend a special game or event because of their limitations, you could offer to go in their place. Providing dinner for the family or an offer to do the weekly shopping could also be helpful.

Everyone I spoke to agreed that an offer to take them to appointments, pick up medications, mow, or rake the yard, was very much appreciated.

Someone who lives alone may appreciate you simply bringing a movie over and watching it with them. They may enjoy playing a board game or simply having someone to talk to.

Those people who have pets may appreciate an offer to walk the dog or possibly do some pet-sitting.

Many people said that others brought gift baskets. One person indicated that a simple gift basket of personal care items including a package of thank you cards and stamps was what she valued most. The cards allowed her the opportunity to thank those who had offered help and support.

Keep in mind that many types of cancer require extensive chemotherapy and oftentimes surgery. Chemotherapy can leave the patient feeling fatigued or sick. Surgery can impede their mobility and leave them with restrictions regarding lifting. Stopping by with bottled water or making an offer to simply do daily household chores might be helpful. One woman said that when she returned home from surgery, she would have appreciated someone coming over to vacuum and put the dishes in the dishwasher.

Sending cards is always a kind gesture. When Allan was first diagnosed, a woman whom I had worked with, who personally experienced a cancer diagnosis, sent inspirational cards on a very consistent basis. Picking up the mail made my day brighter, knowing simply that someone was thinking of us. Sometimes that's all it takes to put a bright spot in someone's day.

These are a few ideas and they are certainly not unique. They are simple acts of kindness that can really make a difference to someone trying to grasp the fact that they have cancer.

So rather than saying, "Please let me know," try saying, "Would it be helpful if I..."

Don't stop believing,

17. Defining a Clinical Trial and Dispelling Common Misconceptions

Many patients and their caregivers contemplate whether they should participate in a clinical trial. Understanding what a clinical trial actually is and dispelling myths regarding what to expect is the crux of this essay.

After combing through many resources related to clinical trials I came upon information from PBS.org entitled *Myths and Facts About Cancer Clinical Trials*. I think it clearly defines the meaning of a clinical trial and addresses the issue of some misconceptions. Hopefully, this information will help patients and their caregivers make an informed decision.

First, what exactly are clinical trials?

Clinical trials are the link between laboratory discoveries and new cancer therapies. They offer patients access to the best cancer care available, while helping researchers find better ways to prevent and treat the disease.

A clinical trial is a medical research study in which people volunteer to test new methods of prevention, screening, diagnosis, and treatment. Because of the importance of clinical trials in cancer treatment, all patients need to be aware that without cancer clinical trials, there would be no treatment advances.

> **A clinical trial is a medical research study in which people volunteer to test new methods of prevention, screening, diagnosis, and treatment.**

Yet misconceptions persist, keeping many patients from learning more about clinical trials. Here are some common misconceptions and facts about clinical trials.

Myth: Clinical trials treat patients like "guinea pigs."

Fact: Patients enrolled in a cancer clinical trial receive either the best treatment currently available or a new, and possibly more effective, therapy. In other words, it is very important that patients understand that their participation in a clinical trial affords them, at minimum, the standard of treatment that they would otherwise receive. Participation in a clinical trial ensures that a patient's health care is closely monitored by leading physicians, and they receive ongoing updates and information as part of the clinical trial process. In addition, the informed consent, which patients read and sign before enrolling, details everything from treatment procedures to potential risks and benefits.

Myth: Clinical trials are a last resort when all other treatments have failed.

Fact: This is a common misconception. In reality, cancer clinical trials exist for all types and stages of cancer, as well as for cancer prevention.

Myth: Clinical trials are too risky.

Fact: There are risks involved, just as there are with any procedure that addresses a life-threatening illness. Your physician can help assess all the factors and determine whether a clinical trial is the best option for you.

Myth: If you enroll in a clinical trial, you may receive a "sugar pill" and get no treatment at all.

Fact: Placebos, or "sugar pills," are never used in place of treatment when an existing standard therapy is available. When you enroll in a trial, you receive either the best treatment currently known for your cancer, or a new, and possibly more effective, therapy.

Myth: Clinical trials test unproven treatments.

Fact: New treatments for cancer—in fact, for any disease—go through a long process of evaluation. All treatments first undergo pre-clinical testing in laboratories. This testing, which does not involve patients, helps identify treatments that may not be effective or that could have intolerable side effects. If the treatment passes the pre-clinical testing phase, it moves into clinical trials, and through three or more phases:

Phase 1: Evaluates safety
Phase 2: Assesses whether the drug will be effective
Phase 3: Determines whether the treatment will be better than the current treatments available

Myth: Health insurance will not cover the costs of a clinical trial.

Fact: Many insurers cover the normal costs of treatment in cancer clinical trials, and many states have mandatory coverage. Check with your doctor or insurance plan to see if you are covered.

Deciding whether or not to participate in a clinical trial is a very personal choice. I hope that the information provided in this post will help both the patient and the caregiver make a more knowledgeable decision based on their specific diagnosis.

Don't stop believing.

18. Resources to Help with the High Cost of Medications

Recently there have been numerous articles in the press about the high costs of cancer medications. For many patients, particularly those who have inadequate health insurance, the cost of cancer treatment can be prohibitive. In the May 15, 2013 edition of *Health Affairs*, researchers at Seattle's Fred Hutchinson Cancer Research Center reported that cancer patients were two and a half times more likely to declare bankruptcy than individuals without cancer. Even for patients who have health insurance, the cost of their co-pays can be high.

Patients and caregivers have enough to worry about without the added burden of figuring out how to pay for life-saving treatments. The task of maneuvering through the financial issues often falls on the shoulders of the caregiver. If you find yourself struggling with this challenge, hope is available for those who qualify. The organizations listed below provide resources that you may find beneficial.

> **Patients and caregivers have enough to worry about without the added burden of figuring out how to pay for life-saving treatments. The task of maneuvering through the financial issues often falls on the shoulders of the caregiver.**

The first place to start is at your own cancer treatment center. Most major cancer hospitals have a financial assistance program, staffed by financial counselors, who can help patients and caregivers explore their options. The financial counselors can help you locate resources that you may qualify for and can help you fill out the paperwork to apply for support.

Organizations such as the Leukemia and Lymphoma Society also have programs to assist patients and their families who do not have adequate insurance coverage to pay for their prescription drug costs. These organizations may also be able to assist with the high costs of stem cell transplants.

Major pharmaceutical manufacturers often have programs where they provide free or reduced-cost prescriptions for those who can't afford them. To find out if the pharmaceutical company that produces the medications you or your loved one is taking, contact the manufacturers patient support department. You could also go to their website and put "financial assistance" in the search engine.

RxAssist, a patient assistance resource center, has a searchable database where you can find out which pharmaceutical companies have assistance programs. To be eligible for such programs, families have to meet income guidelines.

The *Partnership for Prescription Assistance* helps qualifying patients who do not have prescription drug coverage get the medications they need free or at a low cost. Their website also has a searchable database where you can find out what medications are covered. They also have a tool to help you locate free and low-cost clinics in your geographic area.

The *Patient Advocate Foundation* provides direct financial assistance to qualifying patients, who have insurance, to assist them with their prescription drug co-pays. The foundation's counselors work with patients and caregivers to expedite the application process. Payments can be made directly to physicians, pharmacies, or the patient.

Patient Services Inc. assists patients with chronic illnesses by helping them with the costs of insurance premiums and copayments. Patients who qualify may also be eligible for assistance with the costs of other aspects of their care, such as transportation.

Together Rx Access assists patients and families who do not have prescription drug insurance in accessing savings on their medications at their local pharmacy. This website also provides information and links to programs offered by pharmaceutical companies, as well as other resources.

The *Healthwell Foundation* helps patients living with chronic illnesses pay for prescription drug copayments, deductibles, and health insurance premiums. It will help Medicare patients with the costs of premiums for supplemental insurance. The Healthwell Foundation is partnered with the MMRF and other cancer-related organizations.

Provided below are the websites for the resources mentioned in this post. Dealing with a cancer diagnosis is already riddled with anxiety. If you are experiencing issues related to finances, please do not hesitate to ask for assistance. The prime focus of a patient or caregiver is to ensure that you receive the best medical care possible, regardless of your economic status. Everyone is entitled to quality medical care.

Resources:

Healthwell Foundation
https://www.healthwellfoundation.org/fund/multiple-myeloma-medicare-access/

Leukemia and Lymphoma Society
http://www.lls.org/support/financial-support/other-financial-aid

RxAssist http://www.rxassist.org/

Partnership for Prescription Assistance https://www.pparx.org/

Patient Advocate Foundation https://www.copays.org/

Patient Services, Inc.
https://www.patientservicesinc.org/Patients/Types-Of-Assistance

Together Rx Access http://www.togetherrxacces.com/

For more information about these and other resources that provide financial assistance with all aspects of a patient's treatment, see the MMRF's webpage on caregiver self-care and financial support at https://www.themmrf.org/caregiver-self-care-and-financial-support/.

Don't stop believing.

19. Hold That Thought

As I look back over the last nine years since Allan was diagnosed with multiple myeloma, I realize how much that journey has evolved and changed our lives. For me, that evolution can be summed up in four key phrases that I have used to guide and help me. These phrases helped me to not only deal with my husband's cancer, but also have shaped my life and define who I think I am today. What I find interesting is that I did not set out to find an inspirational slogan to hold onto during the challenging times of diagnosis and treatment, but it only recently occurred to me that, in fact, I had. I thought I might share my guiding principles in hopes of helping other caregivers and family members find those rays of light that encourage you to breathe deeply and press forward through what at times seems a daunting task.

> What I find interesting is that I did not set out to find an inspirational slogan to hold onto during the challenging times of diagnosis and treatment, but it only recently occurred to me that, in fact, I had.

When faced with the initial overwhelming shock of the myeloma diagnosis, I clung to the phrase, *"Life is not waiting for the storm to pass, it's about learning to dance in the rain."* I am not even sure where I found or heard those words, but the impact of what they meant truly resonated with me. So rather than being consumed by all the unknowns that had now entered our lives, Allan and I accepted the fact that myeloma was part of the hand we had been dealt and we needed not only to acknowledge it but embrace it. We could not let it define our lives. We both felt strongly that we needed to not dwell on the "Why us?" Rather, we focused our attention on moving forward, finding the positive facets in our lives. I won't say it was always easy, but for us it played a critical role in how we dealt with the situation.

As Allan began his initial treatment of radiation and chemotherapy, we approached each treatment regimen one step at a time. We never got ahead of ourselves, we never said, "But what if?" As I look back, it marked the next phase of the journey with the simple statement of taking *one day at a time*. I pause as I write this because getting ahead of myself and pondering all the "what ifs" was part of who I was. I am not sure why I suddenly was able to adopt this new philosophy of dealing with only one thing at a time, but somehow, I did. As I reflect on it now, it probably is my greatest accomplishment. Even now, when things become challenging I stay focused on the task at hand and deal with it accordingly.

When the decision was made for Allan to undergo the process of a stem cell transplant, I received a message from a dear friend. Simply put, it said, *"Sending you strength, courage and the never-ending gift of hope."* I still hold on to that expression and continue to let it guide me. I think that it sums up the heart of what every patient, caregiver and family member needs in order to keep moving forward. It is a message I freely share with others in the hope that they too, will find both comfort and inspiration. For that reason, we have chosen it as the title of this book.

Lastly, and clearly the most valuable statement that Allan and I live by and truly adhere to the meaning of, is *"Carpe Diem" — Seize the Day, and trust no tomorrows*. I have included that message in some of my essays, but I believe that it is more than a phrase, more than an expression, it is what should govern our actions each and every day. Life holds no guarantees for anyone. If we do not live every day to its fullest we will never be afforded the opportunity to get that time back. It is something Allan and I ponder and reflect on as we greet each new day. While many days pose struggles and challenges for those with multiple myeloma, for us every day is a gift. We strongly believe that we are closer to a cure and that is a thought we continue to hold on to.

Don't stop believing.

20. Suggestions for Taking Care of Yourself

During the celebratory times of holiday seasons, many caregivers tell me that often they feel additional stress. While they look forward to enjoying time with family and friends the increased demand on their time causes some degree of anxiety.

The tips included in this chapter come from suggestions given to a caregivers group at the Dana-Farber Cancer Institute in Boston as well as some from The National Institute of Cancer's website. These tips are not new or unique, but I think, as a caregiver, they are important to ponder particularly at this time of year.

> These tips are not new or unique, but I think, as a caregiver, they are important to ponder particularly at this time of year.

Pay attention to your needs. When you are emotionally and physically healthy, you're likely to be a better caregiver. Identify ways to get rest, exercise, eat a balanced diet, and maintain some connection with others.

Don't be afraid to ask for help. While it may be hard to ask for help, family members and friends are often eager to offer assistance. Accept it, and don't shy away from delegating specific tasks, such as picking children up at school, getting groceries, or driving your loved one to an appointment.

Share. Consider joining a support group, or talking with a fellow caregiver, your family, or friends. You'll benefit from talking about your challenges and stresses with someone who understands. If you need to, consult a social worker or counselor who can help ease your tensions.

Get organized and plan ahead. Keep appointments and contacts organized to help reduce your daily stress, and make sure important documents such as insurance forms are handy. It's also helpful to discuss potentially challenging medical, legal, and financial issues, such as health care proxies, power of attorney forms, and concerns about the future, with your loved one early, before they may be needed.

Work together. You aren't on your own: Your loved one has an entire care team, and they can be invaluable resources for both of you. Ask doctors and nurses about how to manage side effects or talk to a nutritionist about healthy eating for you and your loved one. Never hesitate to ask questions.

Stay close. You and your loved one are in this together, and cancer doesn't have to overpower your relationship. It's important to set aside "cancer-free" time for the two of you, whether that's making dinner together, watching a movie, or just talking.

Watch for signs of exhaustion. Being focused on your loved one can make it easy to miss signs of burn out. Keep an eye out for the emotional and physical signs of caregiver stress, which may include: weight loss or gain; trouble sleeping; and feeling depressed, anxious, irritable, guilty, or inadequate. If you experience these, see your doctor or talk to someone at the cancer center to find ways to reduce stress and maintain your own health.

Learn more about cancer. Understanding your cancer patient's medical situation can make you feel more confident and in control. It may help you to know what to expect during treatment, such as the tests and procedures that will be done, as well as the side effects that will result.

Look for the positive. It can be hard finding positive moments when you're busy caregiving. It also can be hard to adjust to your role as a caregiver. Caregivers say that looking for the good things in life and feeling gratitude help them feel better. Remember that it is important to continue to find the humorous things in life. It is important to laugh. In fact, it's healthy. Laughter releases tension and makes you feel better.

Lastly, caregivers need to allow themselves time to simply "breathe." Everything does not need to be done today. Take time to enjoy every holiday season.

Don't stop believing,

Part IV: The Promise of the Future: A Reason for Hope

1. It's Time to Act

When Allan's oncologist said that he had multiple myeloma, it felt like the floor beneath us had collapsed. He realized our fear immediately and quickly told us of all the advancements that had been made in the previous few years. He explained that multiple myeloma could now be treated as a chronic disease and assured us that it was likely that after some intensive treatment Allan would live a long, near-normal life. So far, he's been right.

As we discussed Allan's options, the oncologist also warned us to not use the internet to get information. He explained that much of the health information on the internet, particularly as it related to multiple myeloma, was either outdated or just plain wrong. Knowing that we would probably not heed his advice, he gave us a couple of safe sites that we could use for reliable information. One of those was the MMRF.

We found a wealth of accurate information on the MMRF's web site. We learned exactly what multiple myeloma is. We also found information about treatment options and clinical trials. The information we found assured us that the treatment protocol Allan's doctor recommended, Revlimid, Velcade, and dexamethasone was state of the art. We discovered that this protocol had been developed with support from the MMRF. More importantly, we also learned that if this did not work, there were other options and even several other promising drugs in the pipeline.

Over the years, we have participated in many educational programs sponsored by the MMRF. In addition to attending patient and caregiver summits, we sign up for webinars and teleconferences that are held throughout the year. These provide information on the latest research and promising new treatments. Research into multiple myeloma is progressing so rapidly that, as one presenter said at one of these seminars, "What we told you last year is now ancient history." Participating in these programs always gives us more hope.

Another great feature of the MMRF's web site is their newly-initiated CoMMunity Gateway. The CoMMunity Gateway is an online forum where patients and caregivers can share information about their experiences, ask questions, and get support. Topics discussed include fatigue, neuropathy, remission, stem cell transplants, and other treatments. The site is moderated by experts who provide their own insight into these issues. In addition, the CoMMunity Gateway is a source of information about clinical trials and the latest treatments. Participating in the CoMMunity Gateway is an excellent way to stay abreast of what is happening in the field.

Early on in our journey through myeloma, we decided that we wanted to do something to give back. We found a few volunteer opportunities at the Dana-Farber Cancer Institute, but we also wanted to do something to help raise funds for future research specifically targeted to multiple myeloma. Again, we turned to the MMRF. We discovered that each year they hold a fundraising event in Boston known as the Race for Research (now the Team for Cures 5K Walk/Run). We decided to form a team.

Initially we were a team of two, but the team grew rapidly. Our first new team member was Allan's former colleague who had lost her husband to multiple myeloma more than two decades earlier. We were also joined by several friends, family members, and former colleagues. Each year the team has grown as has the amount of money we raise. We are now proud of the fact that several other patients and caregivers have joined with us. Our team isn't the largest and we don't raise the most money, but we have made a substantial contribution. While the contribution of one individual or team may not seem like much, collectively many teams and individuals can raise a significant amount of money. In Boston alone in 2017 we raised over $700,000. Similar amounts are raised in several other cities throughout the U.S.

Why is it so important for us to help raise these funds? Very simply, government funding for medical research is not enough. Despite recent increases and President Obama's Moonshot initiative to cure cancer, more funding is needed if we hope for a cure in our lifetimes. We can respond to that in one of two ways: We can sit around and shake our heads and complain about

> **Why is it so important for us to help raise these funds? Very simply, government funding for medical research is not enough.**

how awful it is that there isn't sufficient funding, or we can do something about it. We can stand up and help organizations such as the MMRF raise funds to make sure the research continues. We cannot sit around and wait for someone else to do it for us. We, as patients and caregivers, must do it ourselves.

Right now, the MMRF needs funding to support several new clinical trials that hold the promise of extending the lives of those of us who have multiple myeloma. These cannot be opened without adequate funding. While several new drugs have gotten FDA approval in the past few years, we still do not have a cure. Researchers are currently investigating new classes of drugs, and new treatment options, such as turning on the immune system to fight cancer, that have great potential. Again, this research cannot continue without sufficient funding. These researchers are working hard for us. We need to do something to help them. Researchers feel that they are on the right path. What they need most is more dollars.

If you are not already doing something, consider participating in the MMRF's Team for Cures 5K Walk/Run by joining a team, or forming your own team. If you are not able to participate in the walk, or if there isn't one in your area, there are other ways you can raise funds for research. For example, you can set up a tribute page on the MMRF's web site and ask friends and colleagues to donate.

We know that asking friends and family for donations is not easy. We were a bit shy about it ourselves, but we've gotten over it. We've found that people are very generous. When people hear of your illness they want to do something. What could be better than contributing to the research that will eventually lead to a cure? After all, the future of research depends on it.

Don't stop believing. Life is good.

2. 2015 Was a Very Good Year

Generally favorable weather conditions in wine growing regions meant that 2015 was a good year for wine. It was also an unprecedented year for multiple myeloma researchers. In 2015 four new drugs for treating multiple myeloma were approved by the Food and Drug Administration. That makes it a fantastic year for patients and their caregivers even if they are not wine drinkers.

> **In 2015 four new drugs for treating multiple myeloma were approved by the Food and Drug Administration.**

The FDA approved Farydak in February. Then in November it granted approval for three new drugs to treat patients with multiple myeloma: Darzalex, Ninlaro, and Empliciti. Although these drugs have been approved specifically for use with patients who have become resistant to other therapies, they represent an important breakthrough in the quest to extend the lives of all patients.

Farydak, whose chemical name is panobinostat, is the first of a type of drug known as HDAC inhibitors to be approved by the FDA for the treatment of multiple myeloma. It works by interfering with the activity of enzymes known as histone deacetylases (HDACs), slowing the progression of myeloma and even causing cancerous cells to die. It is approved for patients who have received at least two prior therapies and is used in combination with bortezomib and dexamethasone.

Darzalex, also referred to as daratumumab, and Empliciti, or elotuzumab, are the first of a promising class of drugs known as monoclonal antibodies developed to treat multiple myeloma. Monoclonal antibody drugs identify myeloma cells through specific proteins on the cells' surface. They then either signal the patient's immune system to attack the myeloma cells, attack the cancerous cells themselves, or both. These two drugs were also approved for patients who have received prior treatments, providing additional options for those who have become resistant to other therapies. Both are also being studied for use in combination with other therapies.

Ninlaro, also known as ixazomib, is the first oral proteasome inhibitor. It is in the same class of drugs as Velcade (bortezomib) and Kyprolis (carfilzomib). It has been approved for use in combination with Revlimid (lenalidomide) and dexamethasone. Unlike Velcade and Kyprolis which must be injected, Ninlaro comes in pill form and is taken once a week.

So, what does all this mean for multiple myeloma patients? This is especially good news for relapse/refractory patients who may no longer be responding to other therapies. In clinical trials, many patients achieved significant remissions from these drugs. Thus, for some patients, these drugs are potentially life-saving. For patients who are currently in remission, and don't need these new therapies now, it is reassuring to know that these options are available if and when you do relapse.

The class of drugs known as monoclonal antibodies is very promising. At this writing, they are approved only for relapse/refractory patients, but with further study, they may eventually be available as upfront treatments or for maintenance. In that respect, they have the potential to result in longer and deeper remissions for patients. And, if they can be used in the early stages of disease development, such as with patients who have smoldering myeloma, they may even be curative.

Most importantly, however, the development and approval of these drugs brings us several steps closer to a cure. While the approval of these drugs is important, the fact that many more are in the pipeline is even more important. Breakthroughs are being made all the time. Later in this section we write about several new medications that are currently in the pipeline.

While the approval of these new therapies represents a major breakthrough, they are not cures, and they may not result in sustained remissions for all patients. Other options are still needed, particularly for those who have difficult-to-treat forms of myeloma or who are in advanced stages of the disease. It is critical for the research to continue.

Yes, 2015 was a very good year for multiple myeloma. This New Year's Eve we are planning to celebrate another year of good health with a nice bottle of wine. We think we'll give the 2015 vintage a try. If it's anything like the 2015 myeloma year, it's going to be spectacular.

Don't stop believing. Life is good.

3. Trying to Keep It Simple

In a conversation with Deb about the complexity of medications offered to myeloma patients, another caregiver expressed her feeling of being overwhelmed by the information, especially considering all the newly approved drugs. This conversation gave us the idea for this chapter.

We know in the beginning, it is confusing to try to remember which drug belongs to which class, let alone remember its brand name versus its generic name, how it's administered, and of course how it works. For that reason, we thought that if we could compile all that information in simple chart form it would be easier for patients and caregivers to manage.

With that in mind we created a chart listing the most commonly-used medications. It is our hope that you find it helpful.

Brand Name	Generic Name	How It Works	How It is Administered	Comments
Alkylating Agents				
Alkeran	Melphalan	Slows and stops cancer cell growth	IV, or oral	Often given prior to stem cell transplant
Evomela	Melphalan Hydrochloride	Slows and stops cancer cell growth	IV	New form of melphalan used for conditioning prior to stem cell transplant or palliative treatment
Cytoxan	Cyclophosphamide	Halts cancer cell division, thus slowing or stopping cell growth	IV, injection, or oral	Often given prior to stem cell transplant

Anthracycline Antibiotic				
Doxil	Doxorubicin	Damages DNA in myeloma cells, causing them to die	Injection	Used in combination with Velcade; Being studied in other combinations
Steroid				
Decadron	Dexamethasone	Kills myeloma cells, makes other drugs work better	Oral, injection, or IV	Used in combination with other medications
Immunomodulatory Drugs				
Thalomid	Thalidomide	Causes myeloma cell death; Stimulates the immune system	Oral	Used in combination with several other drugs such as Velcade, Alkeran, and Decadron
Revlimid	Lenalidomide	Causes myeloma cell death; Stimulates the immune system; Affects blood vessels and other substances that feed myeloma cell growth	Oral	Used in combination with other drugs such as Velcade and Decadron

Pomalyst	Pomalidomide	Causes myeloma cell death; Stimulates the immune system; Affects blood vessels and other substances that feed myeloma cell growth	Oral	Used in combination with Decadron, being studied in other combinations
Monoclonal Antibodies				
Darzalex	Daratumumab	Signals the immune system to attack myeloma cells	IV	Currently being studied in combination with other agents
Empliciti	Elotumumab	Activates immune cells to kill myeloma cells	IV	Used in combination with other drugs such as Revlimid and Decadron
Histone Deacetylase Inhibitor				
Farydak	Panobinostat	Slows the progression of myeloma and causes cancer cells to die	Oral	Used in combination with other drugs such as Velcade and Decadron

Proteasome Inhibitors				
Velcade	Bortezomib	Inhibits the growth and survival of myeloma cells, leading to cell death	IV, or injection	Used in combination with Decadron and other myeloma drugs such as Revlimid and Cytoxan
Kyprolis	Carfilzomib	Disrupts processes related to the growth and survival of cancer cells	IV	Used in combination with other drugs such as Revlimid and Decadron
Ninlaro	Ixazomib	Disrupts the myeloma cell's ability to survive by interfering with protein metabolism	Oral	Used in combination with other drugs such as Revlimid and Decadron

Although many myeloma medications seem to work in similar ways, there are differences. For that reason, each patient's myeloma is treated based on the characteristics of the individual's disease and response to treatment. If you have any questions about any of these medications, or your own treatment plan, you should consult your medical team.

Don't stop believing. Life is good.

Sources
American Cancer Society
Celegene Corporation
International Myeloma Foundation
Millennium: The Takeda Oncology Company
Multiple Myeloma Research Foundation

Myeloma Beacon
Spectrum Pharmaceuticals
2015 Multiple Myeloma Patient Education Symposium, Dana-Farber
 Cancer Institute, Boston, MA

4. What's in the Pipeline?

It is never a good time to have multiple myeloma. However, those of us who have it do so in a time of unprecedented progress in treating our disease. We have more hope today than patients in the past.

In a previous chapter, we wrote about four new drugs that gained Food and Drug Administration (FDA) approval to treat multiple myeloma in 2015. While these newly-approved agents give new hope to many myeloma patients, unfortunately they have not brought about sustained remissions in all cases. The good news, however, is that researchers are still hard at work developing and evaluating new drugs. In this chapter, we review several promising new medications that are currently in clinical trials, either alone or in combination with other drugs.

Each of the medications now in clinical trials presents many treatment options since they can, and usually are, combined with other already-approved drugs. It is important to have many options since patients who relapse or become refractory to one treatment, often respond to another. By the same token, because the side effects of various drugs differ, when side effects become intolerable a switch to another agent may provide relief and a better quality of life.

> **It is important to have many options since patients who relapse or become refractory to one treatment, often respond to another.**

Unless otherwise noted, the clinical trials for the drugs listed here are open to relapse/refractory patients. If you are interested in clinical trials investigating these agents, you can use the MMRF's clinical trials tool at https://www.themmrf.org/living-with-multiple-myeloma/clinical-trials-finder/ or the IMF's clinical trials matrix at https://www.myeloma.org/matrix to find more information. Since they are being evaluated in various combinations with other drugs, several trials are ongoing for most of these medications.

Proteasome Inhibitors work by preventing the breakdown of protein in cancer cells, causing their death. Velcade, Kyprolis, and Ninlaro are proteasome inhibitors that are FDA approved for the treatment of multiple myeloma. Several proteasome inhibitors are currently in clinical trials. One that is noteworthy is Marizomib, an IV-administered therapy derived from marine life that has shown promising results in early trials. It may have fewer side effects than other proteasome inhibitors and may work where the others have become refractory. Another is Oprozomib, an orally-administered agent similar in structure to Kyprolis, but since it comes in pill form may be more convenient and provides a possibility for maintenance therapy. While still in early trials, Oprozomib has been given orphan drug status by the FDA. This classification is given to treatments geared toward rare disorders.

Immune Checkpoint Inhibitors. The human immune system usually can tell the difference between normal and foreign cells in the body. By doing so, it can attack the foreign cells while leaving the normal cells alone. It does this by using checkpoints, or molecules on the immune cells that need to be activated or inactivated for the immune system to respond. Cancer cells are sometimes able to use these checkpoints to prevent the immune system from attacking them. Drugs are now being developed to target these checkpoints.

An exciting type of checkpoint inhibitors, known as **Monoclonal Antibodies,** work by stimulating a person's own immune system to attack and destroy cancer cells. Two monoclonal antibodies, Darzalex and Empliciti, were given FDA approval in 2015 but several others are in the experimental stage. Isatuximab (SAR650984) is currently being studied as a single agent in phase III clinical trials and in combination with other drugs such as Pomalyst and dexamethasone. It may work in cases where other monoclonal antibodies do not, providing oncologists with one more tool for relapse/refractory patients. Sylvant (siltuximab) is currently approved by the FDA for the treatment of Castleman's disease, a rare, but noncancerous, disorder of lymph nodes and surrounding tissue. Sylvant has shown encouraging results in early trials with patients with relapse/refractory myeloma. It is also being evaluated in patients with high-risk smoldering myeloma. Miltuzumab, an anti-CD-74 monoclonal antibody, has received orphan drug status from the FDA.

In 2017 the FDA designated a **Humanized Monoclonal Antibody,** currently known as GSK2857916, as a breakthrough therapy for multiple myeloma patients who have failed at least three prior lines of therapy, including an anti-CD38 inhibitor, a proteasome inhibitor, and an immunomodulatory agent. At this writing this drug is in Phase I trials but has shown promise and has been given orphan drug status for the treatment of multiple myeloma.

Keytruda (pembrolizumab), a **PD-1 inhibitor** is currently FDA-approved for the treatment of metastatic melanoma and lung cancers but has been studied for use in other cancers, including myeloma. Despite early trials providing encouraging results when combined with other myeloma drugs such as Revlimid and dexamethasone, the FDA has placed a hold on these trials due to safety concerns. Opdivo (nivolumab), another PD-1 inhibitor, has been approved to treat forms of lung cancer, melanoma, and lymphoma. It is currently being studied in combination with Darzalex and Pomalyst to treat multiple myeloma. Imfinzi (durvalumab), a **PD-L1 inhibitor**, is being investigated as a possible treatment for hematological malignancies, including myeloma. Another PD-L1 inhibitor, Tencentriq (atezolizumab), is approved for treating certain types of solid tumors, but is currently in phase I trials for treating patients with asymptomatic myeloma. Phase I trials using Tencentriq in combination with Darzalex are ongoing.

Another new class of medications, **Histone Deacetylase Inhibitors**, work by increasing the production of proteins that slow the division of cancer cells and cause them to die. One such agent, Farydak, was approved by the FDA in 2015. A promising new drug in this class is Ricolinostat a selective oral histone deacetylase inhibitor. Although it is in the early stages of clinical trials, it has shown a substantial disease response.

Kinase Inhibitors, a new class of drugs for the treatment of myeloma, block the actions of enzymes that help cells grow and divide. In some cancers, these enzymes are too active or are found at high levels and blocking them can prevent cancer cell growth. Inbruvica (ibrutnib), a tyrosine-kinase inhibitor FDA-approved to treat other blood cancers, is currently being studied in combination with other drugs for the treatment of multiple myeloma. It has shown promising results in early trials. Masitinib is an oral tyrosine-kinase inhibitor currently used to treat tumors in animals. It is being studied for use in myeloma in both the U.S.

and Europe. Dinaciclib inhibits cyclin-dependent kinases and has shown an anti-myeloma effect.

Selective Inhibitor of Nuclear Exports block the ability of cancer cells to export tumor suppressor proteins. Selinexor is an oral drug in a new class of agents that inhibit a protein found in cancer cells, resulting in the death of those cells while sparing normal cells. It also suppresses the growth of cancer cells. It has shown encouraging results in treating relapse/refractory patients and has been designated by the FDA as an orphan drug, putting it on a fast track for approval. It is also being studied in various combinations with other myeloma drugs such as Revlimid or Pomalyst and dexamethasone.

Other Chemotherapy Agents are also being investigated for use with myeloma patients. Treanda (bendamustine) is an alkylating agent currently approved to treat other blood cancers. It is thought that it works by damaging the DNA of cancer cells. Much of the current research is taking place in Europe but the MMRF is facilitating trials in the U.S. Aplidin (plitidepsin) is an acyclic peptide anti-tumor agent that appears to have an anti-myeloma effect, particularly when used with other drugs, such as Velcade or dexamethasone.

Chimeric Antigen Receptor T-Cell therapy (CAR-T), an approach that has been used with some success in other blood cancers, is also being evaluated for use with myeloma patients. It falls into the broader class of immunotherapies but uses altered T cells to treat cancer. T cells are white blood cells that are an essential component of our immune systems. In CAR-T therapy a patient's T cells are harvested, genetically altered to attack the cancer, and then reinfused. Early studies have shown that CAR-T therapy may be highly effective in treating advanced multiple myeloma.

BCL-2 Inhibitors. The BCL-2 gene plays a role in cell survival. A damaged BCL-2 gene has been identified as a cause of some cancers and a cause for resistance to cancer treatments. A BCL-2 inhibitor, Venclexta (venetoclax), has been approved by the FDA for the treatment of chronic lymphocytic leukemia. In phase I clinical trials Venclexta has shown acceptable safety and a clear anti-myeloma effect. It shows promise for treating myeloma patients who have translocations, but more study is needed. Clinical trials using Venclexta, Velcade, and dexamethasone are ongoing.

Tasquinimod, an **immunomodulatory, anti-metastatic, and anti-angiogenic agent** has been classified by the FDA as an orphan drug. Although it is being tested for the treatment of solid tumors, early evidence from animal tests suggests that Tasquinimod may be effective in treating multiple myeloma.

Preclinical trials have shown that Viracept (nelfinavir), an antiretroviral drug used to treat HIV, can kill myeloma cells, particularly those that have become resistant to Velcade and Kyprolis; it may also enhance the effectiveness of those drugs. It is also being studied to see if it can restore the effect of Revlimid.

The above list does not represent all the numerous drugs that are now in development. In fact, so many new drugs are being developed, and so much new research is being conducted, that his list is already out of date. Many are still early in clinical trials, but those listed here show promise and are worth watching.

Life is good. Don't stop believing. A cure is coming.

5. Paying it Forward: Why We Volunteer

As we write this, we have just returned from an invigorating and inspiring, weekend volunteering at the finish line of the Pan Mass Challenge (PMC) in Provincetown, MA. We spent the weekend helping unload trucks, setting up tables and chairs, feeding the riders and their families, clearing tables, emptying trash, and then packing everything away again. We are physically tired, but we know that it what we did was nothing compared to what the riders have endured.

The PMC is an annual 192-mile bike-a-thon to raise funds for the Dana-Farber Cancer Institute in Boston. In 2017 6,200 riders and 4,000 volunteers came together to reach a goal of raising over $51 million. Funds raised go for patient care as well as cancer research. Since its founding in 1980, the PMC has raised over to $598 million.

As we journeyed home Monday morning we reflected on why we volunteer. The simple answer, and the one we usually give when asked, is that we want to pay back, in some small way, for all that has been done for us. How can we ever pay back the doctors, nurses, and medical technicians who saved Allan's life? How can we pay back organizations such as the MMRF who sponsored and funded the research that resulted in the treatments that put him in remission? We can't. But we can try.

For us, volunteering is much more than just paying back. When we help to raise funds by participating in the PMC, the MMRF's Team for Cures 5K Walk/Run, the Jimmy Fund Walk, and many other fundraising events, we are helping to raise much needed donations toward finding a cure. We do this in the hope that in the future other people will not have to face the challenges of cancer.

We participate in fundraising activities with the full knowledge that other people before us participated in similar activities to raise the money that funded the research we have benefitted from. As we pay back, we also pay it forward. The money we help raise may or

> **We participate in fundraising activities with the full knowledge that other people before us participated in similar activities to raise the money that funded the research we have benefitted from.**

may not benefit us, but it will benefit others in the future in the same way that the past efforts of others helped us.

Fundraising is not all that we do. We are also involved in several activities that support cancer patients as they are being treated. One of the most rewarding activities that we are involved in is Dana-Farber's One-to-One program where we support and encourage newly diagnosed multiple myeloma patients and caregivers as they navigate through the various stages of their treatment. Having newly diagnosed patients or their caregivers tell you that you made them feel better, or helped to alleviate their fear, gives you great satisfaction.

As part of another wonderful project, we help distribute gift bags to patients who are getting chemo. As we pass out the gifts, we spend a few minutes talking to each patient. When you give patients, who are connected to their IVs a small gift and an encouraging word, the smiles you see on their faces are priceless.

But it's not just about what we do for others. Volunteering also does something positive for us.

When you get a cancer diagnosis you feel helpless. You want to do something to fight back. When we volunteer, we feel that we are doing just that – we are fighting back. We are looking at cancer and saying, "You may have hurt us, but you won't defeat us."

Much of the reason we continue to volunteer is because of the people we have met along the way. We have developed lasting friendships with many who continue to enrich our lives. Their amazing stories of determination and ever-lasting hope not only inspire us but make our dedication to what we do even more important.

In a world where we are frequently exposed to negativity, our volunteer work enables us to see the other side of human nature. The side that thinks not of themselves first, but of others. Volunteers understand that by working together we can face challenges, knowing that we can overcome obstacles and make a difference. As individuals, we might make a small difference, but collectively we can make a huge difference.

So, what is it that makes volunteering so special? To paraphrase a friend of ours who is a cancer survivor and volunteer, it is the camaraderie and community, the sense of vision and purpose, the emergence of the best of humanity, the collaborative approach toward a common goal, the importance of each individual, the diversity of people of all backgrounds working together, the leveraging of strengths, the sense of belonging, the inspiration, the spirit, and the fun.

In our previous careers in education, we felt that teaching defined who we were. We worked hard, took our profession very seriously and were proud of what we did. In some ways upon retiring, we weren't sure that we could find that same fulfillment, yet as we reflect on our volunteer work over the last several years, we couldn't feel more rewarded.

Everyone needs a reason to get up in the morning. Our volunteer work gives us that reason.

Don't stop believing. Life is good.

6. Cancer Moonshot – Progress and Promise

During his last State of the Union address President Obama announced a comprehensive initiative to cure cancer, led by Vice President Biden. Now known as the Cancer Moonshot, this initiative challenged the federal government to step up its efforts to prevent, diagnose, and treat cancer by coordinating and financially supporting the science that will lead to a cure for cancer

In October 2016, Vice President Biden submitted an initial report to President Obama about the findings and plans of the task force formed as part of the Cancer Moonshot. We had the privilege and honor of being in the audience when the Vice President outlined the report in an address given to leading oncologists, researchers, and pharmaceutical company executives at the Edward M. Kennedy Institute in Boston a few days later.

Vice President Biden was confident that the war on cancer, started by President Nixon in 1971, can finally be won because we now have the resources, technology, support, and commitment to do just that. Specifically, we can now hope for a cure because

- There is more collaboration across research disciplines than ever before,
- Technological advances enable researchers to analyze cancer genes and proteins,
- Cancer cells can now be targeted and treated with therapies that boost the immune system while doing less damage to healthy cells,
- An unprecedented amount and diversity of data is being generated via genomics, family history records, lifestyle measurements, and treatment outcomes,
- The availability of computer analysis will allow researchers to use that data to find answers.

Much was accomplished by the task force in its first year. Vice President Biden and the task force have brought many government agencies together to combine their resources to better meet the challenge of improving outcomes for cancer patients. In addition, private sector collaborations were formed to spur new innovations in biomedical research.

The National Institutes of Health (NIH) launched a new partnership of pharmaceutical companies, research centers, foundations, and philanthropies to collaborate on early research. The National Cancer Institute (NCI), which is part of NIH initiated a new public/private partnership with pharmaceutical and biotechnology companies to allow researchers to more easily license and test existing drugs in new combinations that have the potential to cure cancers. NCI also developed a new dashboard on their website to make it easier for patients and doctors to find clinical trials.

To speed up the process of getting new therapies to patients, the Patent and Trademark Office launched an accelerated program to reduce by half the time it now takes to review patent applications for new therapies. The Food and Drug Administration created a center to maximize the review of cancer-related applications to further accelerate making new therapies available. The Centers for Disease Control and Prevention increased its efforts to promote cancer vaccines.

Challenges still exited, however, but the Vice President saw them as opportunities. His task force recommended that in the future the Cancer Moonshot address the following barriers:

- Structures that encourage and reward individual success rather than collaboration,
- Poor recruitment and retention of participants in clinical trials,
- A lack of open access and rapid sharing of research results and data,
- Obstacles in sharing of medical records,
- Slow dissemination of new discoveries, diagnostics, clinical trials, and treatments.

To continue to move forward and improve patient outcomes, the Vice President and the task force have developed a strategic plan for future administrations to follow. The key goals of that plan are

- Catalyze new scientific breakthroughs

1. Strengthen interactions among agencies and engage additional partners in support of multidisciplinary basic cancer research,
2. Expand the implementation of mobile devices and wearable technologies for cancer diagnosis and treatment,
3. Create a high-quality performance status tracking system for cancer patients during therapy and long-term follow-up,
- Unleash the power of data
  1. Rapidly analyze the molecular profile of thousands of tumors,
  2. Create a shared resource of linked clinical datasets,
  3. Improve the clinical data available for research by creating a tool that converts narrative into standardized data,
  4. Advance secure and scalable platforms for data and metadata management for sharing and analysis,
  5. Develop predictive computer algorithms to rapidly develop, test, and validate predictive preclinical models,
  6. Build collaborative relationships with the private sector and academia,
  7. Create a knowledgeable, sustainable, and agile biomedical data science workforce,
- Accelerate bringing new therapies to patients
  1. Modernize eligibility criteria for clinical trials,
  2. Pilot large sample trials,
  3. Develop site/tissue agnostic trials and broaden indications,
  4. Increase the usage of common control and expansion cohort trials,
  5. Achieve greater interaction with pharmaceutical sponsors on international trials,
  6. Create a pilot program for oncology products that utilize real-world evidence,
  7. Strengthen the quality of intellectual property rights to invest in innovation,
- Strengthen prevention and diagnosis

1. Improve HPV vaccination rates in the United States,
2. Implement smoking cessation strategies across the Medicaid population,
3. Screen environmental chemicals through high-throughput in vitro assays,
4. Expand colorectal cancer screening efforts in the United States,
5. Remove barriers that limit access to colorectal cancer screening,
- Improve patient access and care
  1. Identify and implement culturally and linguistically appropriate cancer education and outreach efforts,
  2. Require expedited coverage decisions for patients with a cancer diagnosis in the VA system,
  3. Comprehensively identify cancer survivorship issues and develop solutions to improve health for cancer survivors,
  4. Map cancer service delivery and care across the Nation,
  5. Improve access to care by leveraging technology such as virtual networks.

To accomplish these goals, Vice President Biden recommended that future efforts be focused on the following areas:

- Realign the incentives in the research system,
- Enhance prevention and screening efforts,
- Engage patients as partners in research,
- Expand access to care,
- Create new financial models to improve development of an access to new therapies while addressing the issue of rising drug prices.

The Cancer Moonshot has great promise. But that promise cannot be fulfilled without proper funding, both now and in the future. We, as patients and caregivers, must do our part to make sure that the activities outlined in the task force's blueprint are funded. We must insist that our elected officials make the Cancer Moonshot a priority in future budgets by providing the funding needed to accomplish its goals. The Cancer Moonshot does not rely entirely on public funds, but rather, its success will depend on a combination of public and private funds. We can help here as well by doing our part to raise funds through organizations such as the MMRF.

> We, as patients and caregivers, must do our part to make sure that the activities outlined in the task force's blueprint are funded.

As the task force stated, "The time is now. Together, we can end cancer as we know it." Now is the time to get involved.

Life is good. Don't stop believing.

Sources:

Cancer Moonshot: Report to the President from the Vice President. October 17, 2016. Available at https://www.whitehouse.gov/sites/default/files/docs/finalvp_exec_report_10-17-16final_3.pdf

Cancer Moonshot: Report of the Cancer Moonshot Task Force. October 17, 2016. Available at https://www.whitehouse.gov/sites/default/files/docs/final_cancer_moonshot_task_force_report_1.pdf

7. Survival Day

Each year we celebrate many special events. We commemorate birthdays, wedding anniversaries and holidays. We also note important milestones in the lives of friends and family. Those of us with cancer celebrate Cancer Survivors Day on the first Sunday in June.

In July of each year, we celebrate the anniversary of Allan's successful stem cell transplant. To us, this is our own personal cancer survival day. While the stem cell transplant was only one part of his total treatment regimen, we feel that it was the most important. We looked at it as being the final stage in a very long journey. For us, it was the step that would put him into a long-term remission, where he remains today.

> In July of each year, we celebrate the anniversary of Allan's successful stem cell transplant. To us, this is our own personal cancer survival day.

While we continue to celebrate Allan's actual birthday in February, we look upon the anniversary date of the stem cell transplant as his new birthday. The date observes a rebirth in essence. It is the day we were afforded the opportunity to start over. We realize that not everyone is as fortunate as we have been, so it is a time for us to reflect on those things that we are most thankful for.

Life. We not only celebrate the extra time Allan has been given because of his successful treatment, but we celebrate life itself. Those of you who have been reading these essays know that Allan always signs off with "Life is good." We were both privileged to have had very meaningful lives to begin with, but our lives during the past few years have been even better. Through our volunteer efforts at Dana-Farber Cancer Institute in Boston, we have had the honor of meeting extraordinary patients and caregivers who inspire us and give new meaning to the words strength, courage perseverance, and most important, hope.

Family, friends, and support team. We all appreciate our family and friends. But when faced with a crisis, we realize how important they really are. When Allan was diagnosed, those we were close to rallied around and gave us the support we needed. Simple things, like getting encouraging cards, meant so much. Our family and friends continue to support us. This is most evident every year when they rally around to support us in the annual fundraising walk for the Multiple Myeloma Research Foundation's Team for Cures. In 2017, our team of 53 walkers and runners joined us to raise over $25,000 to help support research toward finding a cure.

Medical team. By medical team, we refer to all our doctors, nurse practitioners, nurses, and medical technicians, not just the oncology group. We are very grateful for everyone from Allan's primary care physician to all his specialists. Allan could not have a better medical team. The thing we appreciate most about his team is that all of them have learned as much as they can about myeloma so that they can better treat him. He is alive today because of them. He also has excellent quality of life because they not only manage his myeloma but are very aware of how the treatment of myeloma impacts other health issues as well.

Myeloma researchers. Where would we be if not for those amazing people who have dedicated their lives to finding a cure for multiple myeloma? Ten years ago, most of the drugs that are standard treatment today for myeloma did not exist. The life expectancy of myeloma patients has tripled since Allan was first diagnosed over nine years ago. Their countless hours of research have been a major factor in Allan's treatment protocol.

The MMRF and IMF. Most of the advances that have come about in the past decade were driven by the Multiple Myeloma Research Foundation, the International Myeloma Foundation, and the research initiatives they have supported. Most importantly, the MMRF pioneered a research model that stresses collaboration instead of competition. This collaborative model has allowed for the advancements in the treatments available today. The MMRF's insistence on researchers working together and sharing information has fueled the progress not only of managing multiple myeloma, but relentlessly moving toward a cure. The IMF has linked researchers from around the world to share their discoveries. Notably, its Black Swan Initiative is dedicated to finding a cure.

Other multiple myeloma survivors. The community of multiple myeloma survivors and their caregivers gives us hope and encouragement every day. The support, compassion and friendship they provide is difficult to adequately put into words. There is a special bond among us, perhaps because we know that we are all in this together. Facing the challenges of a cancer diagnosis is challenging but knowing that you are not alone provides you with reassurance and comfort.

Each other. We have gone through this journey together. From the beginning, we have been a team. Like any team, we have shared the good times and the tough times. This has given us strength and has helped both of us realize how fortunate we are.

Life is good. And it gets better every day. So, don't stop believing.

The Promise of the Future

Part V: Tributes

1. People Come into Your Life for a Reason, a Season or a Lifetime

When you figure out which one it is, you will know what to do for each person.

When someone is in your life for a REASON. . .
It is usually to meet a need you have expressed.
They have come to assist you through a difficulty,
to provide you with guidance and support,
to aid you physically, emotionally, or spiritually.
They may seem like a godsend, and they are!
They are there for the reason you need them to be.
Then, without any wrongdoing on your part,
or at an inconvenient time, this person will say
or do something to bring the relationship to an end.
Sometimes they die.
Sometimes they walk away.
Sometimes they act up and force you to take a stand.
What we must realize is that our need has been met,
our desire fulfilled, their work is done.
The prayer you sent up has been answered.
And now it is time to move on.

Then people come into your life for a SEASON....
Because your turn has come to share, grow, or learn.
They bring you an experience of peace, or make you laugh.
They may teach you something you have never done.
They usually give you an unbelievable amount of joy.
Believe it! It is real! But, only for a season.

LIFETIME relationships teach you lifetime lessons:
Things you must build upon in order to have
a solid emotional foundation.
Your job is to accept the lesson, love the person,
and put what you have learned to use in all
other relationships and areas of your life.
It is said that love is blind but friendship is clairvoyant.

Unknown Author

On the following pages, we pay tribute to people who have come into our lives for a reason, a season, or a lifetime and have helped us along in our journey of strength, courage, and the never-ending gift of hope.

2. People Who Have Come into My Life

A few years ago, a friend of mine, who had lost his wife to cancer, shared the poem in the previous chapter, *People Come into Your Life for a Reason, a Season, or a Lifetime*. The poem, by an unknown author, teaches us that people do not come into our lives by accident, but rather, there is a purpose for their being there. And sometimes, when that purpose has been fulfilled, they move on. Several people have come into my life during my journey with multiple myeloma for a reason and a season and are now gone. But they have left their mark. In this chapter I pay tribute to them.

> **Several people have come into my life during my journey with multiple myeloma for a reason and a season and are now gone. But they have left their mark.**

One of the first people I encountered in my journey was a wonderful IV nurse named Jen. Jen realized quickly that I did not particularly relish having an IV needle inserted into a vein in my hand. Perhaps it was the expression of pain on my face or the way I clenched my teeth. Maybe it was just the look of fear. Jen decided that it might be easier for me if she used a needle that was normally used for infants. The "baby needle" as she called it, made things much easier. Although there were two IV nurses in the office, Jen always made sure that she got to me first. She even stayed with me one day for eleven straight hours when I needed some high dose chemo prior to my stem cell transplant.

During my chemo sessions, my wife and I got to know Jen quite well. She was studying to become a nurse practitioner and she talked to us about her classes and her hopes for the future. Even after my initial treatment was finished I continued to need maintenance therapy. Part of that was the IV administration of a bisphosphonate, a bone strengthening drug. My reliance on Jen continued during this phase. But, one day Jen finished her program, graduated, became an NP, and got a job in a family physician's office.

It's o.k. Jen, I'm doing fine now. And I don't even dread needles anymore. Well, maybe a little bit.

A second person was a fellow patient named Betty. In her long life Betty had been through much, but in spite of all that she had experienced, she remained positive. Betty gave me a coin that was inscribed "I not only believe in miracles, I expect them." Betty was a fighter. She was a bit feisty and could be a bit rough around the edges. But she was an inspiration.

Betty always jokingly referred to me as her boyfriend and Deb as her boyfriend's wife. In addition to seeing each other at the oncologist's office, we periodically talked on the phone and laughed a lot. Betty constantly challenged me to never give up. Sadly, my dear friend has passed away.

It's o.k. Betty, I'm doing fine now. And I promise I'll never give up.

A third person was my nurse practitioner, Melissa. Melissa got me through the initial phases of my chemo and even checked on me when I was in the hospital for my stem cell transplant. After the transplant, I saw Melissa almost every month for six years while I was on maintenance medication. During those visits, she went over my blood work, gave me a mini-physical, and spent time just chatting with us. We laughed a lot and she was always encouraging. During that time, Melissa did take a couple of leaves of absence for the birth of her two children, but she always came back.

Then one day I got a letter from Melissa informing her patients that she had accepted another position closer to home. It was like getting a "Dear John" letter. I was heartbroken. I had lost another very important person who had come into my life. During my journey, I saw Melissa more than all my other medical specialists combined and had really come to rely on her. A couple of weeks after getting Melissa's letter my oncologists decided that I no longer needed the maintenance meds because of how well I was doing, and I also no longer needed to come in for monthly check-ups.

It's o.k. Melissa, I'm doing fine now. And I will continue to do fine because of you.

Many people have come into my life for a reason, a season, or a lifetime and I am better off because of them. I will never forget any of them and I will always be grateful for what they have done for me.

[Update: Shortly after this essay was written, Jen returned to my oncologist's office as an NP to replace Melissa. So, people who may have come into your life for a reason and a season may return for another reason and a season.]

Life is good.

3. My Unsung Heroes

In the previous chapter Allan wrote about a few people who made a huge difference during his journey with multiple myeloma. In his essay, he referenced the poem that opens this section, *People Come into Your Life for a Reason, a Season, or a Lifetime*. The poem suggests that people do not come into your life by accident, but rather, there is a purpose for their being there. Many of those people were important to both of us, some had a particular impact on Allan, and others were very special to me. I would like to pay homage to some of those special people.

There are many incredible people that have made this journey much easier, so where should I begin? Obviously, the remarkable doctors and nurses who provided not only exceptional medical care, but honest and heartfelt opinions as to what we needed to do, are only the beginning of a very long list.

As I began to think about all the people I feel deeply indebted to, I decided to write about a group of people who probably have no idea how much they impacted my life in particular. I refer to them as my unsung heroes.

My unsung heroes came into my life on our first visit to Dana-Farber Cancer Institute in Boston.

Since I have an aversion to parking garages I always use the valet services. As I pulled into the garage for the first time, feeling apprehensive regarding the outcome of the day that lay ahead of us, several attendants were lined up patiently waiting to take our car. We were immediately greeted by one of the attendants with a welcoming smile and a genuine concern for how we were. He rushed to hold the door open for us and told us that he hoped our day went well.

What struck me about the interaction was the fact that he was not simply being polite and courteous, but that he really cared about us. His thoughtfulness showed a true empathy for why we were there and what we were about to encounter. Our first impression

> **His thoughtfulness showed a true empathy for why we were there and what we were about to encounter.**

of Dana-Farber as a place of not only top-rated medical care, but a place of understanding and compassion began with that first interaction in the garage.

On subsequent visits to Dana-Farber the same welcoming attitude was clearly evident each time we entered the garage. The attendants instantly recognized our car. They inquired as to how we had been since our last appointment and again expressed their concern. This simple act of kindness at a time when you feel so fragile was not only welcomed, but truly appreciated.

The true magnitude of what my unsung heroes do on a daily basis came when Allan was hospitalized for a stem cell transplant. Noticing that I now entered the garage alone, the attendants inquired about Allan. I remember telling them that Allan was about to undergo a stem cell transplant, and that I would be coming in every day for the next three weeks. With true compassion, they expressed their well-wishes for a speedy recovery.

The sincerity with which the attendants greeted me each morning as I entered the garage and when I returned in the evening will always hold a special place in my heart. They provided comfort and reassurance in their warm smiles and well-wishes. Before I left each evening, they checked on Allan's progress. I gave them daily reports and we counted down the days remaining in his stay together. They added a bright spot to every day. Their daily acts of kindness are too numerous to put in this chapter, but one that will resonate with me forever, came on the day when Allan was released from the hospital.

On that day, rather than being escorted in a wheelchair to the car, Allan insisted on walking over to the parking garage with me. As we crossed the street from the hospital to the garage, the attendants were all lined up in their red shirts looking highly professional as they always do. Upon seeing us they held their hands high in the air and cheered enthusiastically as we approached the garage. As we got closer, their excitement grew into loud congratulatory wishes. There were hugs and handshakes. Some may view this as a simple gesture, but to me it typified how important the kindness of people we encounter along this journey can be. They initially were strangers who understood the challenges we faced but quickly became an important part of our care team.

I will always treasure the memory of that day.

So, I salute my unsung heroes and I hope that they know what an amazing first and lasting impression they make on all patients and families. They are a credit to their profession and I am grateful that they came into my life.

They keep me believing.

4. A Tribute to Pat Killingsworth

We lost a friend in 2016. Pat Killingsworth was a fellow patient, blogger, and advocate. Pat was the voice of the experienced patient – one who had relapsed and become refractory to standard treatments.

We never met Pat and didn't know him personally. Nevertheless, we always thought of him as a friend. We got to know him from reading his blogs and following him on his own journey through multiple myeloma. He gave us knowledge and shared his innermost thoughts with us. Most of all, he gave us hope.

We always admired Pat for his stamina and his belief that a cure was just around the corner. To say that Pat was a fighter is an understatement. During his journey, he had setbacks, but he was always willing to try everything his doctors could give him, including multiple stem cell transplants, in the belief that he just had to hang on until that cure was found. During World War II Winston Churchill, in an address at his former school, advised students to "never, never, never give up!" Pat epitomized that quote. He never did give up. In fact, he captioned his last blog, written just a couple of days before he died, "I'm not dead yet!"

Pat's posts on both the MMRF's *CoMMunity Gateway* and the *Myeloma Beacon* provided us with much inspiration. As we followed him on his journey we rejoiced when he met success and worried when he had setbacks. We were thrilled when, just a week before he passed away, he reported that a recent PET scan showed no sign of myeloma anywhere. Thus, we were shocked to hear that just days later he contracted pneumonia, his kidneys had failed and that he was not doing well at all.

Multiple myeloma patients and their caregivers form a very special community. Perhaps it's because we all have a shared experience that we have developed a close comradery. Perhaps it's the knowledge that we are all dealing with an incurable cancer that gives us a close bond. We all celebrate when we hear that one of us has overcome obstacles and beaten the odds. Pat gave us many reasons to hope as he fought back after he relapsed.

As a multiple myeloma community, we all mourn Pat's passing. We have not only lost a fellow patient, but we have also lost an important advocate and teacher. Even though Pat is no longer with us he will continue to be an inspiration and a beacon of hope.

Pat taught us that life is good, and that we should never stop believing. He signed off on all his posts with "Feel good and keep smiling!" We will continue to live by those words.

> **Pat taught us that life is good, and that we should never stop believing.**

We offer our deepest sympathy to Pat's family and thank them for sharing him with us.

Life is good. Don't stop believing. Feel good and keep smiling.

5. This One's for You Joe

On May 1, 2016, the MMRF's Team for Cures 5K Walk/Run was held in Boston. As you may know from reading the essays in this book, Allan and I are united in our commitment to the race. For the previous seven years our team, Team Snug Harbor, grew both in size and in the amount of funds raised for the walk. While we are proud of our efforts, it is clearly not just about our team. It is about the 106 teams and individual participants as well. In total, we were 2,500 strong.

The goal for the Boston area for the 2016 event was to raise $375,000. We not only exceeded that goal but collectively raised over $544,000. Although in subsequent years that total was exceeded, at that point it was an all-time record!

Eternally grateful does not even begin to express the feeling we have not only for the people who walked or ran on race day, but those thousands of people who made donations. We know that none of this would have been possible without the continued support of family and friends.

Boston's success is due in very large part to the extraordinary efforts of the MMRF staff. Their leadership and organizational skills are exceptional. Not only do they greet everyone with a smile and a heartfelt hug but their understanding and compassion for why we are all there is indescribable. To them we are also deeply indebted.

For us, race day takes on a special meaning; it is more than a walk/run event. In some ways, it's like coming home after being away for an extended time. It is a place where you find comfort, where your story is truly understood and, most important, where strangers have become treasured friends. As we reconnect, we rejoice in one another's triumphs and shed tears in one another's setbacks. We reconfirm our commitment to the cause: To find that elusive cure.

While we always look forward to the excitement of race day, this year's race also took on a very somber note for our team. One of our team members and our good friend, Joe Banish, lost his courageous battle to multiple myeloma. Shortly before race day, Joe and his devoted wife Debby were told that essentially, they were out of treatment options and there was little that could be done to combat the ravages of the disease. I am not sure if I would have had the fortitude to accept that prognosis, but Joe not only accepted it, he remained positive. I don't think that he ever stopped believing.

A true testament to Joe's character was made evident mere weeks before the race. In one of our final conversations with him, he pledged to make this race the best one ever. He set a personal goal of raising $8,000. In the last days of his life he achieved that goal. I cannot think of a more noble gesture.

Even now, after the race is over, I reflect on Joe's words. He did not think of himself, his thoughts were for others—others who continue to wage the battle. He wanted for them what he himself could not attain. In a world where we often forget that it's not all about me, Joe's example needs to resonate with us all.

> He did not think of himself, his thoughts were for others—others who continue to wage the battle.

Recently, I have thought a lot about Joe and how he impacted our lives. I remembered the chapter Allan wrote about people who come into our lives earlier in this section. The idea for the chapter came from a poem entitled *People Come into Your Life for a Reason, a Season or a Lifetime*. I think Joe came into our lives for all three. Although we knew Joe for only a season, I know he came into our lives for a reason. The reason was to inspire us and make us better people. He gave us strength, courage, and the never-ending gift of hope. His friendship and memory will be treasured for a lifetime.

And yes, Joe it was indeed the best race ever.

Don't stop believing.

6. Allan's Medical Team

When we think of all the people who came into our lives during our journey with multiple myeloma, first and foremost on our list are two very special oncologists, Dr. Timothy Ernst and Dr. Edwin Alyea.

When an MRI showed that Allan had something on his spine that looked like a malignant tumor, his primary care physician referred him to a local oncologist, Dr. Timothy Ernst. Dr. Ernst has extensive experience treating blood cancers and was recently cited by *Boston Magazine* as being one of the top oncologists in the metropolitan Boston area.

We had two heart-wrenching days between getting the call from the PCP and the appointment with Dr. Ernst. During that time, we had to return from a trip to Texas and gather Allan's medical records and other information the oncologist would need. As the hours went by the anxiety grew.

Dr. Ernst immediately put us at ease. His kind, gentle manner was very reassuring. As Allan wrote in the first section, Dr. Ernst gave us hope from the start. We left his office that day feeling much better. He gave us the assurance that whatever it was that was showing up on that MRI, it could be treated successfully. He also told us that we would take everything one step at a time.

> **Dr. Ernst immediately put us at ease. His kind, gentle manner was very reassuring.**

Right from the start Dr. Ernst did not let us get ahead of ourselves. When we first met him, he looked Allan in the eyes and said, "You don't have cancer until I say you have cancer." There was something in that statement that stopped the wheels from turning and stopped us from thinking the worst. Instead, for the first time since getting the call from the PCP, we started to have hope and realized that whatever Allan had, we could deal with it.

After many more tests Dr. Ernst told us that Allan did, in fact, have cancer. However, in telling us that he had multiple myeloma he explained that, although incurable, it was a very treatable disease. He gave us the assurance that although the road would be difficult, the outcome would be good. He felt that Allan's prognosis was positive and told us of other patients he had who had survived myeloma for many years.

We had great confidence in Dr. Ernst. He is the kind of healer who sizes up patients quickly and knows exactly how to deal with them. He explained everything to us in detail, answered our questions, but again, never let us get too far ahead of ourselves. Throughout Allan's initial treatment with radiation and chemo, he constantly assured us that everything would be o.k. He gave us the strength and courage to persevere even through the worst of the treatment.

Towards the end of the chemo regimen, Dr. Ernst referred us to Dr. Alyea at the Dana-Farber Cancer Institute in Boston for a consult to see if Allan was a viable candidate for a stem cell transplant. We left that appointment with the procedure scheduled.

Dr. Alyea is a stem cell transplant specialist who is well-known for his research in this area. He is the associate director of the stem cell transplant unit at DFCI and was recently named one of the area's top doctors by *Boston Magazine*. He has confidence in his own abilities as a physician and, in turn we immediately knew that he was the right specialist for us.

> Dr. Alyea is a stem cell transplant specialist who is well-known for his research in this area…. He has confidence in his own abilities as a physician and, in turn we immediately knew that he was the right specialist for us.

Dr. Alyea looked over Allan's records and latest test results and conferred with Dr. Ernst. He explained that even though tests showed that Allan was in remission, since multiple myeloma was incurable he could still have some minimal residual myeloma that did not show up on the tests. He felt that we needed to take advantage of the good results Allan had already obtained by doing everything we could to eliminate that residual myeloma. At this point we discussed in detail the advantages of a stem cell transplant. Since Allan was otherwise healthy and strong, Dr. Alyea felt that he was an excellent candidate for a transplant. We had such faith in his judgment and his skills, we agreed immediately.

We won't say that the transplant was smooth sailing, but Allan's experience was probably typical. Although he had his ups and downs, on balance, it went well. Every time a problem developed, Dr. Alyea was right there to take care of it. The long-term results also could not have been more positive. As of this writing, Allan has enjoyed over nine years of complete remission and we credit much of his success to Dr. Alyea's knowledge and skills.

A transplant is followed by a period of isolation with many dietary restrictions. When it came to those restrictions, Dr. Alyea was very cautious. In fact, during this period we nicknamed him "Dr. No" because any time we prematurely asked if restrictions could be relaxed, his response was a simple, but emphatic, "No." By following Dr. Alyea's guidelines, Allan did remarkably well during the entire recovery period by avoiding infections and other setbacks. We followed Dr. Alyea's advice very carefully, and in the end, it paid off. We will be forever grateful to Dr. No.

Dr. Ernst and Dr. Alyea are backed up by wonderful teams of nurse practitioners, nurses, medical technicians and many other unsung heroes who have also played major roles in Allan's success. It is impossible to name them all, but we are indebted to each and every one of them.

Dr. Ernst and Dr. Alyea continue to monitor Allan's myeloma. They work together as a team and consult with each other before any treatment decisions are made.

Because of them, life is good, and we will never stop believing.

Tributes

APPENDICES

Several years ago, a discount clothing store in the Boston area advertised with the motto "an educated consumer is our best customer." The store's philosophy was that the more the customer knew about clothing, the better the store could serve them. At various seminars that we have attended we have heard many physicians echo this sentiment by stating that their best patients are those who educate themselves about the disease and their treatment options. It is our firm belief that patients and caregivers who take the time to learn everything they can about multiple myeloma and the options available today are in a better position to proactively manage the course of their own treatment. In doing so, they have a better chance of staying healthy and living longer.

Finding reliable information that the layperson can understand is difficult. As we learned early on, the internet is a great source of misinformation and should be used with great caution. Organizations such as the American Cancer Society, The Leukemia and Lymphoma Society, the Multiple Myeloma Research Foundation and the International Myeloma Foundation have produced numerous patient education resources that are reliable and accurate. While these materials are particularly beneficial for newly diagnosed patients and their caregivers, they are also helpful for those who are further along in their journeys. Combined, these materials provide an excellent overview of multiple myeloma and the various treatment options.

In the appendices that follow we have assembled a list of resources that we have found to be invaluable in terms of finding accurate, reliable, up-to-date information about multiple myeloma and treatment options.

Appendices

Appendix 1: Books

Many books have been written in the past few years on various cancer topics including multiple myeloma. We have read several and have found a few that are well worth reading. Here are some of our recommendations. The books listed here are all reasonably priced, some are even free, but the information they contain is priceless.

BOOKS ABOUT CANCER IN GENERAL

***The Emperor of All Maladies: A Biography of Cancer* by Siddhartha Mukherjee, Scribner, 2010.** In this book, which won the Pulitzer Prize for general nonfiction in 2011, Dr. Mukherjee, an oncologist and cancer researcher, archives the history of cancer and the discoveries that have led to today's treatments, and in some cases, cures. Although it is not specifically about multiple myeloma, it is well worth reading for anyone who would like to know more about the discoveries that have been made from the time Sidney Farber first developed the first successful chemotherapy for childhood cancers.

Through this book, we meet the scientists, researchers, doctors, and even patients whose efforts over the years have brought us to the point that many cancers can be cured and others, such as multiple myeloma, can be treated as chronic diseases. Although the book details the science behind the treatments, it is written in terms a layperson can understand.

This book comes in both hardcover and paperback, as well as electronic versions. It was also the subject of a PBS documentary by Ken Burns.

***Everyone's Guide to Cancer Therapy* by Andrew H. Ko, M.D., Malin Dollinger, M.D. and Ernest H. Rosenbaum, M.D., Andrews McMeel Publishing, 5th Edition, 2008.**

Although this book is written by physicians and oncologists, it is intended for the layperson. It is the most authoritative reference guide to cancer we have found. Now in its fifth edition, it offers a comprehensive source of up-to-date information about cancer in general as well as all individual common cancers. the book addresses cancer diagnosis (including recent advancements in assessments) and treatment (including all standard of care therapies). In this respect, it describes what cancer is and provides information about available standard and experimental treatments. In addition, the book has information about other important aspects of cancer treatment such as management and supportive care. Each chapter includes questions that patients should be asking their doctors.

This is not a book that one would sit down and read cover-to-cover. Rather, it best serves as a desk reference that can be used when you need to look up information about a specific cancer.

The current edition is available in paperback and electronic format.

BOOKS ABOUT MULTIPLE MYELOMA

***NCCN Guidelines for Patients: Multiple Myeloma*, National Comprehensive Cancer Network, 2016.** This book, developed by medical personnel from cancer centers that are associated with the National Comprehensive Cancer Network, is the best-written comprehensive guide to multiple myeloma we have seen. It includes up-to-date information about how the disease is diagnosed and treated. It is written in a style that laypersons can easily understand. This book is an essential guide to all who have recently been diagnosed and are beginning to make decisions about their treatment. It is also a valuable reference for those of us who are further along in our journeys.

The book is divided into five parts. The first section provides an overview of multiple myeloma, including symptoms and an explanation of what myeloma is and how it develops. That is followed by an excellent overview of the tests used to diagnose and monitor the disease. The third and fourth parts discuss treatment options and the selection of treatments based on the stage, severity, and type of myeloma. These chapters provide comprehensive information on all options with a thorough synopsis of available drugs. The final section offers some insight for patients deciding which option is best for them. It includes questions you should ask your doctor and advice on weighing your options. The book also includes an excellent glossary.

A print version of the book is available from Amazon but a pdf version, that can be printed or read on a computer or tablet, is available as a free download from the NCCN website.

***The Myeloma Survival Guide: Essential Advice for Patients and Their Loved Ones* by Jim Tamkin and Dave Visel, Demos Health, 2014.** This book is unique in that it is written by a multiple myeloma patient, who also happens to be a physician, and the caregiver of a cancer patient. Several chapters are also written by guest authors who have an expertise in the subject matter of the chapter. Written in a straight-forward, down-to-earth format, this book nevertheless covers some important ground. In addition to chapters about coping with the disease itself, the book includes information on practical matters of dealing with illness. It is divided into three parts. The first part provides basic information about what the patient needs to do when first diagnosed. The second part covers financial matters. It provides advice on dealing with insurance, taxes, personal finances, and workplace issues. The final section reviews various treatment options and offers suggestions on treatment management.

A strength of this book is that it provides detailed information about the various treatments currently available for multiple myeloma patients. It also reviews some of the promising drugs that were in clinical trials at the time, some of which have since received FDA approval. Much of this is provided in chart form that makes it an excellent reference guide. It is a book that newly diagnosed patients and their caregivers will find useful. These chapters will help the patient and caregiver navigate through health care system.

This book is available in paperback and electronic versions.

Books About Personal Journeys Through Cancer

***A Lucky Life Interrupted: A Memoir of Hope* by Tom Brokow, Random House, 2015.** Tom Brokow is best known as the former anchor of NBC's Nightly News. Brokow was diagnosed with multiple myeloma in 2013 after suffering severe back pain. Brokow considers himself to be the luckiest person he knows, but his good luck changed when he received his diagnosis. Nevertheless, he considers the time he spent in treatment to have only been an interruption to an otherwise exciting and fortunate existence. In his book, Brokow chronicles his journey through diagnosis and treatment, while taking some side trips to talk about some important news stories that he covered in his career. He also talks about his family, how much they mean to him, and how their support was so important.

We can all relate to his story, especially as he poignantly writes about his journey and the changes it has made in his life. There were numerous passages that provided perfect descriptions of what Allan had experienced. We found his narrative to be moving and entertaining at the same time. Despite his diagnosis, he is still mindfully aware of how lucky he has been and continues to be. His story is inspiring and one that can give all of us hope. It is well worth reading.

This book is available in both hardcover and paperback. Electronic versions are also available.

***Promise Me Dad: A Year of Hope, Hardship, and Purpose* by Joe Biden, Flatiron Books, 2017.**

This book chronicles Vice President Biden's family's journey from the time his son Beau was diagnosed with glioblastoma through the months after his untimely death. During this period Vice President Biden had to balance the responsibilities he had with his job and his duty to his country with his responsibilities as a husband, father, and grandfather. At this time, he also struggled with the decision of whether he should throw his hat into the ring and run for President. His account of what he did on both the national and international stage as Vice President is interwoven with the heartbreaking story of his son's journey with cancer.

As anyone who has lost a loved one to cancer knows, the journey is replete with hope and joy that is often balanced by fear and sadness as the patient and family experience many ups and downs. Periods where treatments appear to be working bring joy and hope, but that can be offset by periods when the cancer is progressing, bringing disappointment and fear. In this poignant account of how Beau, and the entire Biden family, struggled, the Vice President provides us with insight into what it is like to suffer such a momentous loss. More importantly, in his description of how he personally dealt with his own grief, he provides us with inspiration as he fulfills the promise that he made to Beau that no matter what happened he would be all right.

This book is available in hard cover, paperback, electronic format and as an audiobook read by the Vice President himself.

BOOKS FOR CAREGIVERS AND FAMILIES

Complete Guide to Family Caregiving: The Essential Guide to Cancer Caregiving at Home by Julia A. Bucher, R.N., Ph.D., Peter S. Houts, Ph.D. and Terri Ades, D.N.P, F.N.P-BC, AOCN, American Cancer Society, 2012.

This book, written by practitioners with extensive experience treating cancer patients and their caregivers, is a comprehensive guide for caregivers of newly diagnosed patients' as well as those caregivers who have been managing the challenges that every caregiver faces at some point in the process of patient treatment.

Its step-by-step approach, written in language that is easy to understand for the layperson, is an excellent reference guide. It provides detailed information regarding various cancer treatments, and managing care, both emotional as well as physical, for the patient as well as the caregiver.

It also includes information on dealing with insurance companies, health care providers, and many other situations that may occur while caring for a patient. Its section on "Helping Children Understand" is a must read for any caregiver dealing with the issues that surround talking to children about a cancer diagnosis. The book also contains a resource guide as well as a glossary that all caregivers will find beneficial.

This book is available in paperback and electronic formats.

New Healthy Eating Cookbook **by Jeanne Besser, American Cancer Society, 2016.**

The fourth edition of this book presents the latest scientific evidence regarding diet, exercise, and health. It contains more than 120 new recipes reviewed by the American Cancer Society's medical staff. Each recipe is simple and healthy. The book contains nutritional basics, as well as information that can help the reader make healthy eating choices. It highlights the parts of a healthy diet and what that diet looks like, tips to make cooking at home easier, how to understand food labels, and the importance of portion control.

In addition, the book lists ideas for nutritious snacks and guidance on making healthy choices when eating out. As an added bonus, there is information about simple ways readers can incorporate more exercise into their daily schedules. In its mission to save lives, the American Cancer Society hopes that by sharing what they know they can help people make positive changes in adopting a healthy lifestyle by eating well and exercising.

This book is available in paperback and electronic formats.

Appendix 2: Pamphlets, Brochures, and Booklets

The MMRF has combined several pamphlets into a Patient Toolkit. The following guides are included in the toolkit, which can be ordered at https://www.themmrf.org/living-with-multiple-myeloma/resources/ or by calling 203-652-0441. Individual pamphlets can also be downloaded from this website.

Managing My Myeloma: Resources to Get the Best Care Possible. This brief brochure provides an introduction to the MMRF and the services it offers. It gives an overview of the website, including its tool for finding clinical trials. Further, it offers a synopsis of the support and education resources the MMRF provides, such as their webinars and patient summits.

Multiple Myeloma Disease Overview. This pamphlet begins with an overview of multiple myeloma. It explains what myeloma is and how it affects the patient. The next section addresses the diagnostic process and explains the various tests that are used when myeloma may be suspected. After explaining how the disease is staged, the brochure has a comprehensive section that details the various symptoms and complications of myeloma with detailed information about how each can be addressed to assure quality of life. The booklet contains many charts and diagrams, along with a glossary of terms, that help the layperson better understand its contents.

Multiple Myeloma Treatment Overview. As much as you trust and have confidence in your oncologist, it is important for patients and their caregivers to actively participate in the development of their treatment plan. To do this, patients need to be informed about the various medications and treatment options available today. Further, since treating multiple myeloma often involves several stages, it is important to know about all possibilities. This comprehensive booklet provides an excellent overview of the currently approved drugs, including the side effects that can be anticipated. It also gives a summary of the stem cell transplant process and includes a discussion of maintenance therapy. In addition, it explains the options that are available for patients who have relapsed or have become refractory to their first line of treatment. An important aspect of this booklet is a section on clinical trials. As with the other booklets in the toolkit, it includes several charts and diagrams along with a glossary. In summary, this pamphlet will provide patients and caregivers with the knowledge needed to have an informed discussion with their medical team.

Multiple Myeloma Caregiver Guide. We don't go through this journey alone. Patients have spouses, partners, significant others, children, family members, or friends who assist them and provide important support and care throughout the treatment process. This guide has been developed to provide those caregivers with the information they need as they help patients manage their disease and navigate the treatment options. This booklet is full of practical information to help caregivers better understand the disease and the treatment options. It explains the roles of all members of the medical team and outlines the stages in a standard treatment plan. Importantly, it offers suggestions for caregivers on dealing with the stresses and concerns they inevitably will encounter.

The Path to Precision Medicine in Multiple Myeloma. Multiple myeloma is not one disease, but rather, it has several subtypes. The standard treatment option for one subtype may not be best for another. For that reason, researchers have concentrated on developing precision medicine, a type of therapy that identifies the best course of action based on the patient's individual profile. This brochure explains how precision medicine works and outlines the progress that has been made in this field.

The IMF has numerous pamphlets that deal with specific topics. To order or download any of the guides described below, go to https://www.myeloma.org/publications or call 800-452-2873.

Patient Handbook. This comprehensive booklet provides an overview of multiple myeloma with a focus on diagnosis and treatment options. Illustrated with many charts, diagrams and pictures, this guide delivers detailed summaries of what myeloma is, the stages and types of myeloma, how it is diagnosed, and how it is treated. The booklet includes tables that outline the tests used to diagnose and stage myeloma and describe the drugs that are used to treat the disease.

Concise Review of the Disease and Treatment Options. This booklet, although concise, provides a comprehensive overview of multiple myeloma. It includes sections on the epidemiology, pathophysiology, and clinical features of the disease, as well as current standard treatment options, and new and emerging treatments.

Understanding ... Series. The Understanding Series pamphlets cover every aspect of multiple myeloma including all the drugs approved by the FDA for the treatment of multiple myeloma. Other booklets cover topics such as the treatment of bone disease, clinical trials, various tests used to diagnose multiple myeloma and assess the effects of treatment, stem cell transplants, etc.

The Leukemia & Lymphoma Society publishes many booklets on various aspects of blood cancers that can be downloaded or ordered at http://www.lls.org/resource-center/download-or-order-free-publications. The following two booklets are of particular interest to myeloma patients.

Myeloma. This booklet provides an excellent overview of multiple myeloma. It covers subjects including diagnosis, staging, treatment, complications, side effects, and follow-up care.

Blood and Marrow Stem Cell Transplantation. This booklet gives an overview of transplants for all blood cancers. Although it is not specific to myeloma, anyone facing a stem cell transplant will find it useful. It covers the various types of transplants and explains the process for each.

The National Bone Marrow Transplant Link has numerous resources specifically for patients who have had a bone marrow or stem cell transplant and their caregivers. The booklets below are available through the NBMT Link at www.nbmtlink.org.

***Guide to Bone Marrow and Stem Cell Transplant: What to Expect and How to Move Forward*, by Keren Stronach.** This booklet provides information to guide patients, caregivers and health care professionals through the bone marrow and stem cell transplant process from beginning to end. It includes sections on preparing for the transplant, the steps in the transplant process itself, and what happens after the transplant. It also contains a useful list of resources.

Bone Marrow/Stem Cell Transplant Frequently Asked Questions. This booklet was written for patients, caregivers, and families headed for a bone marrow or stem cell transplant. It is a resource that provides the tools, information, encouragement, and support for both patients and their loved ones throughout the process. Questions, and the answers provided, cover all aspects of the transplant process.

***Survivorship Guide for Bone Marrow/Stem Cell Transplant: Coping with Late Effects*, by Karen Stronach.** More and more patients are long-term survivors of transplants. Once beyond the post-transplant years, survivors have a new set of challenges. Written by a transplant survivor, this booklet is a practical guide for survivors living with late effects. It offers information on many post-transplant topics, such as graft versus host disease (for those who have had an allogeneic transplant), emotional well-being, sexuality and intimacy, work-related issues, and caring for yourself physically.

Caregivers Guide for Bone Marrow/Stem Cell Transplant: Practical Perspectives. Written especially for caregivers, this booklet provides insight into the role caregivers play in the success of transplants. It offers practical advice on dealing with the responsibilities of caregivers and on dealing with the emotional aspects of being a caregiver.

Appendix 3: Websites

The internet can be a valuable source of information. Unfortunately, however, it can also be a source of much misinformation. When Allan was first diagnosed his oncologist warned us about searching the internet for information about multiple myeloma because, in his words, "Most of the information you will find is either outdated or just plain wrong." That does not mean that all websites are suspect, but it does mean that you must be careful. Here are a few that we have found to be reliable and useful.

Multiple Myeloma Research Foundation

https://www.themmrf.org/

International Myeloma Foundation

https://www.myeloma.org/

American Cancer Society

https://www.cancer.org/

Leukemia and Lymphoma Society

http://www.lls.org/

National Cancer Institute

https://www.cancer.gov/

Most major cancer centers also have websites that can be reliable sources of information about multiple myeloma. The list below is certainly not exhaustive but includes those that we have explored and found to be excellent.

Dana-Farber Cancer Institute, Boston, MA

General website: http://www.dana-farber.org/

Multiple myeloma website: http://www.dana-farber.org/multiple-myeloma/

M.D. Anderson Cancer Center, Houston, TX

General website: https://www.mdanderson.org/

Multiple myeloma website: https://www.mdanderson.org/cancer-types/multiple-myeloma.html

Johns Hopkins Medicine, Baltimore, MD

General website: https://www.mdanderson.org/

Multiple myeloma website: https://www.hopkinsmedicine.org/kimmel_cancer_center/types_cancer/multiple_myeloma.html

Memorial Sloan Kettering Cancer Center, New York, NY

General website: https://www.mskcc.org/

Multiple myeloma website: https://www.mskcc.org/cancer-care/types/multiple-myeloma

City of Hope Cancer Center, Duarte, CA

General website: https://www.cityofhope.org/homepage

Multiple myeloma website: https://www.cityofhope.org/myeloma

Appendix 4: Other Resources

The Multiple Myeloma Research Foundation and the International Myeloma Foundation provide a wealth of resources for patient and caregiver information. These include videos, webinars, and patient symposiums. These are made available either free or at a very low cost.

Webinars

Both organizations also offer webinars and teleconferences (generally around one hour in length) on specific topics of interest to patients and caregivers. We have particularly found their updates on the proceedings of the major cancer conferences to be an important way of keeping up to date on the latest research.

IMF: https://www.myeloma.org/understanding/imf-tv/living-well-myeloma

MMRF: https://www.themmrf.org/living-with-multiple-myeloma/education-programs/webinars/

Patient Symposiums

Both organizations also offer patient symposiums in cities throughout the country. These symposiums feature sessions by leading researchers in the field.

IMF: https://www.myeloma.org/patient-and-family-seminar and https://www.myeloma.org/regional-community-workshops

MMRF: https://www.themmrf.org/living-with-multiple-myeloma/education-programs/patient-education/

Videos

Both the MMRF and the IMF have produced videos on various aspects of multiple myeloma. There are far too many for us to list here but we urge you to explore their websites to find more information. Videos of their past webinars and patient symposiums are available.

IMF: https://www.myeloma.org/understanding/imf-tv

MMRF: https://www.themmrf.org/living-with-multiple-myeloma/education-programs/

Appendix 5: Tips for Evaluating Health Sites on the Internet

Earlier in this book we relayed that when Allan was first diagnosed, his oncologist cautioned us about using the internet to find information about multiple myeloma. He gave us a few sites that were reliable. In Appendix 3 we list those sites along with a few others.

We recognize that myeloma patients have other health issues and may need to find reliable information about those conditions. Again, caution should be exercised whenever using the internet for health information. Outdated information is not always removed from internet sites and many sites make misleading, as well as false, claims about products or treatments.

How can you determine if a web site is reliable? Here are a few tips.

Check out who runs the site. The first thing you should do is determine who sponsors the site. Reputable sites will have an "About Us" tab that should provide this information. Sites run by a government agency, a hospital, a medical school, or well-known health organizations can be trusted. Be skeptical of any others. While web sites developed by a company or an individual may be reliable, they also may have a bias or a particular purpose in posting the information. It's best to check further and consult other sources.

Check to see if the site has an editorial or review board. A website that has a process whereby all material is reviewed by a panel of experts is generally reliable. Even so, you should check out the credentials of the expert panel. Are they doctors? What hospitals are they affiliated with?

Evaluate the purpose of the website. Is the site's purpose to provide information or is it trying to sell you something? Many sites are sponsored by companies selling a product. Many sites are run by pharmaceutical companies and these can provide valuable information about their medications. Other commercial sites may be trying to sell you an unproven product. You should always verify the information on company websites by consulting independent sites.

Find out how current the information is. Many web sites include a statement at the bottom of each page stating when it was last reviewed or updated. Others may have a copyright date that will indicate when the page was originally posted. Anything more than one or two years old may not be current and should be consulted with caution. It's better to search for something more current.

Be careful of websites that present opinions rather than facts. The information should be verifiable. Look for references and then check out those references. Beware of opinions that are stated as facts. When opinions are offered they should be identified as such.

Be very skeptical of so-called news sites promoting a product. The Federal Trade Commission has issued warnings about false online news sites that promote products. The sites cited by the FTC often feature a reporter from a news agency writing on the results obtained by users of the product. These sites look legitimate but are actually advertisements for the product and the reporter, news agency, and testimonials may be fabrications. Always read the fine print as this may give you clues as to the real purpose of the site.

Constantly be on the lookout for quackery. Regrettably, unscrupulous individuals use the internet to prey on vulnerable patients. Be skeptical of claims that seem too good to be true or that offer miracle cures. Look for scientific data, not testimonials from other patients. When scientific data is cited, check it out to make sure it is genuine because scam artists often falsely claim that something is backed by scientific research.

Check with your doctor. As an added precaution, you should always ask your doctor about any information you find on the internet.

Appendices

Made in the USA
Monee, IL
02 November 2020